FOWL!

Bird Flu: It's Not What You Think

By Dr. Sherri J. Tenpenny

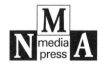

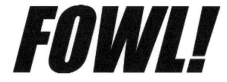

Bird Flu: It's Not What You Think

Copyright © 2006 Dr. Sherri J. Tenpenny

10 9 8 7 6 5 4 3 2

Printed in the United States

ISBN-13: 978-0-9743448-3-6
ISBN-10: 0-9743448-3-4

The truth knocks on the door and you say,
"Go away, I'm looking for the truth," and so it goes away.

Puzzling.

~Robert M. Pirsig
Zen and the Art of Motorcycle Maintenance

DISCLAIMER

All information, data, and material contained or provided herein is for general information and educational purposes only. It reflects the compiled efforts and opinions of the author. It is not intended to be, nor is it construed to be, legal or specific medical advice.

All information and web sites were verified and active as of the date and time the manuscript was sent to the printer. Because web sites are eliminated, modified, or updated frequently, the author assumes no responsibility for the removal or updates of links or references.

The information contained herein reflects the author's opinions at the time of the completion of the manuscript. Information and data will change over time as they become available. Updates and possible corrections will be discussed and/or related through seminars, the web site (www.BirdFluHype.com), and/or other forms of general communication. The author assumes no responsibility for updating information that may modify any information presented herein.

The author, New Medical Awareness Seminars, LLC and OsteoMed II, individually, jointly, and severally, are not responsible for the health of, or the health consequences of, any person as a result of this information or other information produced and distributed by New Medical Awareness Seminars, and/or OsteoMed II.

Acknowledgements

The most important person in bringing this book to life is Cindy Stolten. She must be the most incredible Internet research wizard in the world. Without her assistance, this book would have taken many times longer to write. In addition, writing a book while working with someone online in "real time" who lives in a different state certainly makes the long hours at the keyboard much more enjoyable.

The next three persons to thank are Tris Bolinger, David Dalton, and Debbie Radvar. Tris' steady hand and incredible computer skills created www.BirdFluHype.com almost overnight. From the publishing world and an excellent writer, David helped to add clarity and editorial comment when I was stuck on concepts and feeling lost in the text. Debbie put her marketing hat on and relentlessly pushed me through to completion.

Without the support of the entire OsteoMed II staff, nothing in my life would be possible. You've picked me up when I was tired and discouraged, and you have all played a very significant role in my life, personally and professionally.

Linda Corlett	Cheryl Leuthaeuser, D.O.	Gail Singer
Kirsten Ericson	"Dee Dee" Laff	Chris Speck
Nicole Gordon	Melissa Luby-Hammad	Annette Sylvester
Carol Kilbane	Faith Mann	Clay Walsh, D.O.

I extend gratitude to my dear friends and editors par-excellence, Ingri Cassel and Don Harkins. Don's inspiration started me down the road to the final copy of this book, challenging me to examine the problems we are facing globally and generously imparting his editorial comments. Ingri kept me honest by not letting me hedge on the hard facts. I couldn't have done this without you two.

I am indebted to my closest friends, who have been cheering me on to completion of a book for many years: Lou Paget, Bonnie Shaker, and Sandi Asazawa. Without your encouragement and prodding, the brim of my procrastination hat would still be pulled down over my eyes. Thank you for being there; here's to the books to come.

A few other people need to be mentioned for the support and inspiration they have given me; they know the specifics, and I am grateful they are in my life: Kathi Williams; Dawn Richardson; Stephanie Cave, MD; John Wilson, MD; Doug Moore, PhD; Doris Rapp, MD; Corwyn Beaumont and Dave Block.

A big thanks to my wonderful editor, Norm Friedman. You took a diamond in the rough and turned it into pure gold.

Dedication

To my mom: You've always believed in me and have been my biggest cheerleader. Thank you for all you have done for my entire life.

To my husband Kevin: You make everything in my life worth living. You are my best friend and my inspiration. Your support of me in every way is more than a dream come true. Thank you for making my life so much fun and filling it with so much love.

Special Dedication

To the memory of Nicholas Regush, my friend and my mentor. Thanks for your contribution to this book and all that I write.

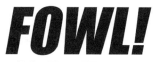

FOWL!
Bird Flu: It's Not What You Think

Foreword

When the hype about bird flu started to draw national and international attention during the spring of 2004, it was difficult for me to comprehend why such a frenzy was being created over so few reported outbreaks and even fewer deaths.

Hysteria should always be looked upon with suspicion; there are logical steps rational minds need to take before declaring the worst-case scenario has arrived. Viewed incrementally, the first steps should be to advise caution, and as the facts become substantiated, alarms and warnings should be introduced. At all cost, panic should be avoided. What would lead national governments and global authorities to abandon a common sense, rational approach to a few deaths, call for international planning, and predict global chaos at the first signs of a virus among flocks of chickens and a handful of people?

Because I have a rather suspicious attitude toward the government in general and the vaccine industry in specific–a way of thinking that has evolved from thousands of hours over many years investigating the problems caused by vaccines–a number of questions crossed my mind early on as I started to search for plausible motivations.

1. Why are so many farm chickens sick? What has made these birds more susceptible to the effects of the H5N1 virus? Why are droves of migratory birds dying in obscure locations across the globe?
2. Who wants all the chickens dead? Whose interests would be most served by elimination of the independent farmer's lifestyle and means for supporting his family?
3. Why are the human cases clustered in Southeast Asia? As the virus appears in other parts of the globe, is there a connection between the reported outbreaks?
4. The vaccine manufacturers always win, but the stakes are higher than usual. What's behind the nearly blank check being handed to them? Or better, *who* is behind it and *why* are they

pushing for mandatory vaccination?
5.   Are global conditions similar to those at the time of the 1918 Great Pandemic?

From those few questions, this story began to unfold. Once I started to look for answers, the truth was hidden in plain sight. When you go to the Land of Oz and pull back the curtain, it is amazing what you find.

Introduction

Writing a book is a daunting task and finding the common thread connecting vaccines, animal rights, the environment, the pernicious objectives of agribusiness and pharmaceutical companies, the vestiges of war, and the agendas of governments seemed at first to be impossible. At one point, the thought of writing several books instead of one book was even entertained. But as the facts accumulated and jelled, the connections between these diverse topics came together with stunning clarity.

The first chapter, "Thinking for Yourself," sets the tone for the rest of the book. You, the reader, are challenged to change your beliefs to something more reasonable than what has been convincingly and authoritatively presented by the media. Chapters 2 and 3 explain what an influenza virus is, how it is named and how a pandemic is said to occur. Some readers will scan this detailed information, and others will savor it.

To put the current pandemic discussion in perspective, Chapter 4 reviews three previous influenza pandemics and offers a different view as to why they occurred.

Chapter 5 discusses the similarity between the feverish planning for a bird flu pandemic and two similar events: the threat of a smallpox outbreak and the swine flu scare. The chapter dispels many misconceptions about smallpox and points out the similarities between the 1976 swine flu program and the occurrence of bird flu today. One frightening difference is that the families of persons injured by the bird flu vaccine will have no recourse against vaccine manufacturers, even if the vaccine causes their relative's demise.

Needing a plan to keep everyone vigilant, Chapter 6, "The New Playbook Arrives" details the 10-step plan engineered by risk communication experts. Understanding this scheme is essential for dissecting news reports as the bird flu drama continues to unfold.

Influenza vaccines are discussed in Chapters 7, 8, and 9. How the vaccine is manufactured, what is in the vaccine and what is planned for the bird flu vaccination programs will help you make an informed decision about injecting flu shots into your body—or the body of your children. Chapter 10 outlines the laws and presidential executive orders that could lead to requirements of mandatory vaccination.

With billions of dollars being spent to stockpile Tamiflu, the drug that is supposed to prevent the spread of bird flu, Chapter 11 explains why Tamiflu won't work and why its use during an influenza outbreak may actually result in resistant "mutant" viruses, resulting in a more serious problem.

Chapter 13, "The Killing Fields," and Chapter 14, "Sick Chicks in the U.S." introduce the impact of agribusiness—especially in Southeast Asia. The annihilation of more than 200 million free-ranging chickens, raised primarily by independent farmers, is causing a socioeconomic strain on already poor populations. The economic interests of the multinational agribusiness companies in the U.S., Thailand, China and India have much to gain from the elimination of local chickens.

Reports of dead migratory birds around the world have led some officials to blame wild birds for the spread of H5N1 but raises the critical question: What is suppressing the immune system of these hearty birds, making them more susceptible to the effects of influenza viruses? The answer, which involved the connection between Agent Orange and unhealthy birds, is discussed in Chapter 15. "Sick Migratory Birds: Canaries in the Coalmines" warns us that the mass culling of our early-warming messengers is akin to shutting off a blaring fire alarm without looking for a fire.

The most significant cluster of human deaths from H5N1 has been in Vietnam. Chapter 16, "Sick Humans," points out that irresponsible environmental contamination, there and around the world, is leading to outbreaks of aggressive viruses. The more contaminated the soil and water are with dioxin, chemicals, nuclear waste, human sewage and industrial filth, the more likely humans will become susceptible to serious consequences from influenza.

Chapter 17, "Tying It All Together," does just that: Bird flu is a wake up call to global chemical contamination. The chapter revisits the 1918 Spanish flu pandemic—linking the deaths to the massive chemical warfare used during World War I and offering evidence that chemicals are contributing to bird flu today. Chemical clean-up, not pandemic planning and massive vaccinations, is what is necessary to stop the next global catastrophe.

"The Activists Playbook," Chapter 18, is a response to the government's playbook detailed in Chapter 6. This chapter offers suggestions for taking an environmental stand and protecting your family against the insidious agendas exploiting the threat of an influenza pandemic.

Community disaster planning is an extraordinarily good idea. Natural disasters can occur anywhere and at any time. Having a plan to deal with food shortages, power outages, and increased healthcare requirements is essential for every city and town. But FOWL! goes far beyond encouraging public planning.

FOWL! affirms the urgency of joining diverse activist groups— environmentalists, animal rights proponents, vaccine awareness groups, anti-war groups and those working to halt the use of genetically modified food. All of these hard working, dedicated alliances are, in their own way, similar to the three blind men trying to describe an elephant. Although there are many versions of this fable, the story goes like this:

> A group of blind men once heard that an extraordinary beast called an elephant had been brought into their village. Resolved to obtain a picture, they put to use the only tool they had: They used their hands to feel the beast. As the three community leaders approached the animal to learn more, one touched its leg, the other a tusk, the third an ear. Believing they knew what the elephant looked like, they returned to their clan to share the news. But when asked to describe what they had learned, each person's description varied widely.

> The one who felt the leg maintained that the elephant was a pillar, extremely rough to the touch, and yet strangely soft. The one who had caught hold of the tusk refuted this description. Describing the elephant

as hard and smooth like a metal post, he proclaimed there was nothing soft or rough about it. The third who had held the ear in his hands said that the elephant was both soft and rough, but was neither a pillar nor a post. His description was that an elephant looked like a broad, thick piece of leather. Each was right to a certain degree; each person communicated the part of the elephant that was in his experience. But none came close to describing—or comprehending— the entire elephant.

Activism occurs much the same way. Each group is intensely focused on their particular part of the elephant. This is not a criticism. Because the issues are complex, funds are often tight, and the number of people doing the day-to-day work is often small, a singular focus is necessary. However, the issues surrounding the bird flu offer a portal for seemingly different groups to unite: *FOWL!* grasps an appreciation for the "whole elephant."

Through *FOWL!*, environmentalists will find they have a lot in common with those who oppose vaccines. People fighting for the rights of farm animals will learn they have unexpected similarities with those fighting to stop war. Veterans and citizens struggling for compensation due to dioxin and Agent Orange poisoning will find surprising parallels with those engaged in the battle to stop the use of genetically modified foods.

It's all the same elephant. We're all in this together.

The pharma-chemical-agribusiness giants are eliminating our choices, contaminating our food, destroying our health and poisoning our planet. What will the next 20 years look like? What will remain for your children and grandchildren? Distinctions and differences will remain, but the time is now to join together with the focus on unity. Strength comes in numbers, and my hope is that millions will join forces through information gleaned from *FOWL!* and we can subjugate this huge beast while there is still time to make a difference.

Fight for your opinions, but do not believe that they
contain the whole truth, or the only truth.
~Charles A. Dana, U.S. Newspaper Editor (1819-1897)

Chapter 1: Thinking For Yourself

Starting points:
- What you need to know
- Thinking for yourself

News reports encouraging the masses to rush to their doctors' offices for their annual flu shots arrive in concentrated clusters. When the big push starts each fall, few are aware this flurry of attention is not due to spontaneous reporting, but due to a coordinated manipulation of the media, sponsored by vaccine manufacturers in conjunction with the Centers for Disease Control and Prevention (CDC) and local health departments.

Vaccination is the primary method for preventing influenza and its severe complications. How many times has that message been used to imprint the "necessity" of the flu vaccine into our collective consciousness? Early in 2004, a presentation given at the National Immunization Program by the associate director for communications at the CDC, Glenn Nowak, PhD, revealed the extent to which the media is used to force consumers into believing in the necessity of the flu shot.

During the week of September 21–28, 2004, according to information provided by Dr. Nowak, the airwaves carried a whopping 1,056 messages—that's approximately one every 15 minutes—urging viewers or listeners to get their flu shots. The most intense reporting on influenza generally starts in early October and extends through mid-February, averaging 200 stories per week for 20 weeks. That's at least 4,000 messages per season. In 2004–2005, the cost of a prime time, 30-second ad on a major network averaged nearly $427,000.[1] Network stories of "flu shot delays" and maps of influenza outbreaks amount to free advertising, with the unspoken subtext being "hurry, get your flu shot." The locations where flu shots can be obtained—such as churches and health departments—on the local evening news adds to a free publicity bonanza for flu vaccine manufacturers. It is obvious that the use of television to promote the use of flu vaccines amounts to *hundreds of millions* of dollars in "free advertising" for the pharmaceutical manufacturers, among the wealthiest companies on earth.

What types of messages are delivered? Here is a partial list, along with the number of times the message pierced the airwaves in 2004:[2]

Message	Number of messages/wk
Doctors recommend/urge flu shot	(285)
The flu kills 36,000 per year	(221)
This could be a bad/serious flu year	(174)
Flu vaccine is the best defense against the flu	(149)
Oct./Nov./Dec. is the best time to get the vaccine	(117)
Now is a good time to get the flu vaccine	(106)

The fear-mongering usually continues throughout the fall, until influenza vaccine sales reach a peak. Then the media hawking subsides as quickly as the melting snow in spring.

Given this level of indoctrination, is it any wonder the average person views the flu vaccine as one of the most important prevention tools for maintaining health? Is there any doubt that the media will be used to promote mass vaccination as the means to prevent the new "influenza pandemic" once the vaccine is available? Is it any wonder that it is difficult to convince people to reconsider their position on the flu shot and get them to understand that the vaccine is not only ineffective, but can actually cause harm?

Research into the way people process media reports sheds some light on the reasons it is difficult for people to change their beliefs, even in light of new, compelling information. A 2003 study by psychologist Professor Stephan Lewandowsky from the University of Western Australia investigated the effects of retractions and disconfirmations on people's memories and beliefs related to the war in Iraq. More than 800 people from three countries—Germany, Australia, and the U.S.—were shown a list of events reported in the media. Some of the events were completely true, some were reported as true and then retracted, and some were complete fabrications. Each study participant indicated whether or not he or she had heard of the event and rated the likelihood of it being true. Then, for each report the individual had recalled hearing, he was asked to note whether it had subsequently been retracted and if the recall changed their feeling about the original report.

The results of the study were both fascinating and telling. The more clearly the Germans and the Australians recalled that an event had been retracted, the less they believed that the original claim had been true. However, if Americans recalled hearing the report, *even once,* they tended to believe it was true even if it had been retracted or denied.[3]

An interview reported in the *Wall Street Journal* with Dr. Lewandowsky explained that people build "mental models" of what they believe is true. He went on to say, "By the time they receive a retraction, the original misinformation has already become integrated into their mental model, or world view, and disregarding it would leave the world [as they know it] in shambles."[4] In other words, Americans will continue to believe something is the truth even after they have been shown the information is false.

The study also supports the formation of what is referred to as "false memories." False memories are constructed by combining actual memories, or information, with new content that is *suggested* by others. Over time, the individual may forget the source of the original information, but with constant repetition, he or she will come to believe the added suggestions are completely true. The more comfortable a person becomes with a particular version of the truth—for example, that vaccines are safe, effective, and cause little harm—the less likely he or she is to question the premise. It appears that people will not trust corrected information—for example, showing proof that a vaccine has not been tested for long-term safety—unless they are already suspicious about the original premise, or something substantial occurs, such as a vaccine injury, to cause them to take another look at their perceived "truth."

According to Lewandowsky's study on Iraqi news events, Americans are the most difficult to convince that what they initially believed is indeed false, even when presented with irrefutable evidence. For example, although no weapons of mass destruction have been discovered, nearly 30 percent of U.S. respondents still believe they exist. "Given that it is in fact not true, given that none have ever been discovered, we would classify those responses as a false memory," says Lewandowsky.[5] It appears Americans accept what they hear at face value, especially if they hear it on the news.

Thinking for yourself

In much the same way, it is difficult to redirect people away from what they have been told and what they have come to believe is true about the coming bird flu. We are told the next global pandemic is about to arrive that will be "the end of Western civilization as we know it," wreaking economic havoc around the world so pervasively that "no person will be untouched." Both television and print media chronicle daily reports to keep us worried and in a state of impending doom.

But what if these proclamations are false?

What if nearly everything you've been hearing about the coming pandemic is incorrect? What if you were presented with an overwhelming amount of information to show that what the media is hyping about the coming pandemic is **not true**? Would you pause and question what you have been hearing on the airwaves? Or would you be part of the 30 percent who will not be convinced, no matter how convincing the argument?

The sudden arrival of unsettling information can impact lives in dramatic and unexpected ways. Studies have shown that the impact of a shocking new discovery is similar to the emotional and psychological jolt that occurs when we are told of the sudden death of a loved one—it is wrenchingly difficult to accept. However, if the news is integrated in stages, such as hearing someone has cancer and has six months to live, it is usually somewhat less distressing. The well-accepted stages of loss, as defined by Dr. Elizabeth Kübler-Ross, offer insights into how deeply information about the coming pandemic has been integrated into our belief system and why disrupting that belief with new information can be so troubling.

Dr. Kübler-Ross' classic book, *On Death and Dying* (1969), presented her theory that people who are dying go through five stages of grief: denial, anger, bargaining, depression, and acceptance. The Kübler-Ross model has been widely adopted and applied to many situations where someone suffers a loss or a sudden change in social identity. The stages are not necessarily sequential or linear in their progression, and some people tend to stay in one stage for longer periods than others. But for most, the stages of the model hold true.

A good example is a discussion about the effectiveness of the flu vaccine. On September 21, 2005, *The New York Times* published a ground-breaking story reporting on a study with strong evidence that flu shots are ineffective and possibly even harmful in the most highly targeted group, the elderly. Published in *The Lancet Online* (9/05), the study provided no new data but reviewed 64 existing studies that evaluated the effectiveness of the flu vaccine over 96 flu seasons. The authors concluded that the effectiveness of the flu shot—*particularly* in the elderly—was "wildly overstated."

"The runaway 100 percent effectiveness that's touted by proponents [of the flu shot] was nowhere to be seen," said Dr. Thomas Jefferson, a Rome-based researcher with the Cochrane Vaccine Fields project, an international consortium of scientists who perform systematic reviews of research data. In addition, Dr. Jefferson went on to say, "What you see is that marketing rules the response to influenza, and scientific evidence comes fourth or fifth. Vaccines may have a role, but they appear to have a modest effect. The best strategy to prevent the illness is to wash your hands."[6]

The reaction to this report was predictable. Many people first denied, and then became angry, over this information. Denial was pervasive among health officials who employed press releases to counter the study and continued to encourage as many elderly people as possible to get the vaccine despite compelling evidence that it doesn't work.[7]

Denials also came from the general public, such as, "Well, the flu shot always protects me." Some proceeded to bargaining by saying, "Shouldn't *some* people get the flu shot?"

Obviously, reversing an ingrained belief about the effectiveness of flu shots is a difficult task, even in light of solid evidence. Many refuse to give up the long-held belief that a flu shot protects them from the flu. Some pass into Kübler-Ross' stage four—acceptance—and with that evolves an entirely new belief. But this time, the new belief is based on scientific research and personal information. It is not based on indoctrination by the media and healthcare providers. This new belief—a different type of "knowing"—is immutable.

When we first discover what we have been told about the bird flu may not be the whole truth, we may deny it (stage 1) and become angry (stage 2). There will no doubt be the feelings of incredulity. Bargaining (stage 3) will come with questions such as "Why would the government lie to us?" or "Well, at least part of what they are saying is true, isn't it?" Giving up the notion that the "government is here to protect me" is a big step that many choose not to take.

An often-repeated quote from writer Dresden James comes to mind:

> *A truth's initial commotion is directly proportional to how deeply the lie was believed. When a well-packaged web of lies has been sold gradually to the masses over generations, the truth will seem utterly preposterous and its speaker a raving lunatic.*

It wasn't the world being round that agitated people, but that the world wasn't flat.

This book is meant to cause a lot of "commotion," and I will likely be considered a "raving lunatic" by some people (by Dresden James' definition, that is). But it is time for Americans to wake up to the deception being promoted through the propagation of false premises by government agencies and the manipulated media. The avian flu scare is just the latest act in an ongoing world government drama.

The hype about the coming pandemic and the avian flu is a recycled drama, rife with government manipulation brought to you courtesy of an obedient media. The obvious beneficiaries are the drug companies. Less apparent, but much more insidious and perverse, are the behind-the-scenes agendas of the huge agribusiness conglomerates and the enormously overlooked problems of agrichemicals and the chemicals of war. Armed with new information based on solid medical, biological, and political truths, a new belief system about vaccines, our government, and our world will emerge.

From the bitterness of disease man
learns the sweetness of health.
~Catalan Proverb

Chapter 2: The Flu As We Know It

Starting points:
- The historical impacts of microbes
- An overview of "the flu"

A strong argument can be made that germs are rulers of the world. Epidemics, inextricably intertwined with the agricultural and industrial revolution, have left their mark on history in cultures around the world. For hundreds of years the effects of germs have played a significant role in the evolution of modern civilization, from the shaping of public policy to the outcome of wars.

In 1566, Holy Roman Emperor Maximillian II and an army of 80,000 prepared to invade Hungary, which was under Turkish domination. The invasion was unsuccessful, not because the Turks were militarily superior, but rather because the Roman ranks were decimated due to a typhus epidemic. Similarly, the Swedes lost control of Russia in 1708 because of the bubonic plague.

In the late 18th and early 19th centuries, Napoleon's greatest adversary was not the British navy. It was microbes. His Russian campaign stands out as a classic example of strategic blundering. Students of history know that the Russian winter proved to be a more implacable enemy than the czar's forces, yet few know that the size of the army had already been whittled down by typhus. Of the

320,000 to 600,000 soldiers (accounts vary dramatically) who left France, 70 percent succumbed to typhus before they reached Moscow. Russians used delaying tactics that weakened the troops and allowed typhus to ravage the remainder of Napoleon's troops even more. Only 50,000 soldiers were left to occupy Russia, and, after the winter, a mere 3,000 returned home to France.

The 19th century saw several other wars where the outcomes were determined as much by diseases as by weapons. During the Crimean War (1854–1856), as an example, ten times as many British soldiers died from dysentery as from Russian bullets.[1]

In the modern history of disease and warfare, World War I particularly stands out. On the heels of the "war to end all wars" came a pandemic—a worldwide outbreak of the relatively benign infection called influenza. History reports that the virus originated in the United States and was carried by soldiers to France. When the war ended and the troops returned home, the Spanish Flu returned home with them. In an effort to halt the spread of the disease, many cities, states, and countries imposed restrictions on mass gatherings and travel. Restaurants, dance halls, and theaters were closed for up to a year. Some communities even outlawed the shaking of hands.[2] But as quickly as it appeared, the virus of the Great Pandemic retreated, leaving deaths and questions in its wake.

The Flu Today

The flu is conventionally defined as a "highly-contagious illness caused by viruses that infect the respiratory tract." Compared with adenovirus, which causes the common cold, influenza viruses are often associated with more severe symptoms. Viruses are thought to spread from person-to-person via respiratory droplets released by coughing and sneezing. The viral particles bind to mucous on the surface of the respiratory tract and then bury themselves into the

Influenza symptoms
• Fever, three to five days
• Headache
• Extreme fatigue
• Nasal discharge
• Shivering
• Dry cough
• Sore throat
• Body aches

cells that line the lungs. Following an incubation period of about 48 hours, flu symptoms abruptly appear.

Of course, a textbook list of symptoms does not quite capture the suffering endured by those who contract the flu in any given year. There's an old joke about the "24-hour bug" that goes something like this: The first 12 hours you're afraid you're going to die, and then for the next 12 hours you feel so uncomfortable you're afraid you might not. As the body goes through the complex physiological process to expel the virus and the contaminated mucous of the lungs, the symptoms can be miserable.

While no one wants to get the flu—even with the quasi-perk of a couple of days off from work or school—the fact remains that most adults and children recover completely within two weeks. Most overtly healthy individuals, *whether living in 1566 or 2006,* will not contract the flu at all.

Scientists should always state the opinions
upon which their facts are based.
~Author Unknown

Chapter 3: The Avian Flu: What You Need to Know

Starting points:
- Influenza viruses are categorized as types A, B, or C. Humans are most affected by influenza type A viruses.
- Two surface proteins, referred to as (H) or (HA) and (N) or (NA), allow influenza viruses to invade cells and also serve as naming devices.
- Highly pathogenic avian viruses have been causing infections for centuries.
- Viruses morph through processes called "drifting" and "shifting."

All influenza viruses are not created equal. Or as George Orwell might point out, some influenza viruses are more equal than others.

Influenza viruses are identified as three distinct immunogenic types—A, B, and C—and a large number of subtypes. Type C viruses are associated with either a very mild respiratory illness or no symptoms at all. They are not associated with epidemics and do not carry with them a public health impact. Influenza type B viruses also tend to be part of minor illnesses. Having a propensity for older persons, influenza type B viruses are most often identified in nursing home outbreaks. Influenza types C and B have not been identified in any species except humans.

Influenza viruses in category "A", known to affect many different species, are divided into subtypes based on different combinations of two surface proteins called antigens. Any foreign substance that enters the bloodstream and stimulates the immune system to produce antibodies is defined as an antigen. The outer shell of influenza A viruses is covered with two types of antigens: One is called hemagglutinin, signified by the abbreviation (H) or (HA), the other is called neuraminidase, identified as (N) or (NA). The differences between the H and the N antigens provide the basis for classifying and naming all the many subtypes of influenza type A viruses.

Fifteen different H antigens (referred to as H1 to H15) and nine different N proteins (referred to as N1 to N9) are commonly known to exist. Another antigenic type, H16, has been identified in some scientific papers, but is not universally accepted.[1] The various combinations of these antigens are the basis for sub-typing, and notably, every possible combination of H and N can be found in wild and domestic birds.

A virus is not a living organism, but it can make copies of itself that can be passed on to other hosts. The ability to replicate is what gives the impression that a virus is "alive". There are only five groups in which influenza A viruses can replicate: large land mammals, sea mammals, wild birds, domestic birds, and humans. Land mammals associated with influenza viruses include swine and horses. Sea mammals encompass seals, dolphins, and whales.

The focus of this book is the association of influenza A viruses with *wild birds*—particularly migratory water birds, geese, and ducks—and *domestic birds* defined as chickens and turkeys raised for slaughter. Since 1977, only a few influenza A viruses, specifically H1N1, H1N2, and H3N2, have been associated with humans.

Even though the official nomenclature for identifying individual viruses is cumbersome and long, the naming system serves as a code for virologists and other researchers to identify different characteristics. For example, the official name of one H5N1 viral subtype is A/chicken/Vietnam/HauGiang/178/2004(H5N1). Breaking it down, the code identifies the virus as an influenza **type**

A virus, isolated from a **chicken** in **Vietnam,** in the city of **HauGiang.** It was the **178th** virus isolated in **2004** of serotype **H5N1.**[2]

The number of different serotypes for H5N1 alone is in the hundreds; The number of antigenically distinct influenza A viruses is in the tens of thousands.[3] The fact that hundreds of subtypes exist for H5N1 influenza virus is more than just a scientific curiosity. As stated by Nancy Cox, PhD, chief of the Influenza Branch, National Center for Infectious Diseases at the CDC, "If we don't get a close match, the vaccine will be less effective, producing illness, hospitalizations, and death."[4] For those who purport the importance of getting a vaccine to protect a person from getting the flu, how can a "close match" be good enough?

Just because a virus is present doesn't mean that it is causing a problem. In fact, influenza A viruses can be completely benign, silent passengers in the intestinal tracts of waterfowl. During trans-global seasonal migration, thousands of ducks and geese congregate in available lakes and ponds along their journey. An examination of the lake water after the flocks have converged would reveal tens of billions of influenza A particles. As many as 130 viral subtypes have been identified in the viral soup. It is this free exchange of genetic material between viruses that has scientists concerned.

Influenza A subtypes have been delineated as either "mildly pathogenic," meaning they cause minimal or no disease, or "highly pathogenic," meaning their presence has been associated with widespread death among all types of birds. All outbreaks of Highly Pathogenic Avian Influenza (HPAI) viruses since the 1980s have been caused by antigen subtypes H5 or H7. For this discussion, these three antigenic types are important to remember.[5] The bird flu virus in the news is a highly pathogenic subtype referred to as H5N1. Unlike what is being portrayed by the media, outbreaks of highly pathogenic viruses are not new; These viruses have been causing problems in bird populations for a very long time.

Old player in a new game

The first highly pathogenic avian influenza virus was isolated on the Italian peninsula in 1878. Like many immigrants of the Ellis Island era, "Fowl Plague," as it became known, reached the shores of the U.S. via New York City sometime in 1924. The initial outbreak, along with another that occurred five years later, was contained through the destruction of the poultry stock in the entire area.

It is presumed that when a highly pathogenic influenza virus is found in a flock, the virus will be transmitted indefinitely through the stool of the birds. Complete destruction of all the birds is considered to be the only option for eradicating the outbreak, even if the birds show no sign of the infection. That practice continues today with the large-scale culling of flocks used to eliminate the presence of the virus.

Records show that since 1959 there have been 21 reported outbreaks of highly pathogenic avian influenza worldwide. The majority have occurred in Europe, with a few emerging in Mexico, Canada and even the U.S. Of the 21 incidents, five resulted in significant losses to regional economies. Minor outbreaks occurred sporadically throughout the U.S. and abroad until 1983, when a major epidemic of highly pathogenic H5N2 appeared on farms in rural Pennsylvania. Two years and $70 million later, the outbreak had been controlled. However, nearly 17 million birds—mostly chickens and domestic ducks—had been destroyed, leading to escalated consumer costs of approximately $350 million, mostly due to a 30 percent jump in retail egg prices.[6]

In another part of the world and nearly 10 years later (2001), H5N1 viruses were isolated at the Western Wholesale Food Market in Hong Kong from geese imported into the central slaughterhouse. Widespread testing was undertaken, and many birds throughout the province were found to be positive, prompting authorities to order the slaughter of virtually all poultry—chickens, ducks, geese, and quail—in the territory. The slaughter cost the farms and markets across the region more than $10 million.[7]

16

Outbreaks of HPAI seem to be occurring more often. In February 2004, an outbreak of H5N2 viruses afflicted poultry on a single farm in Gonzales County, located in south-central Texas. Detected through routine monitoring for the presence of influenza viruses, the affected birds were quarantined and the area was disinfected. The quarantine was lifted March 26, 2004, and after five days, the U.S. Department of Agriculture announced that the Texas outbreak had been completely eradicated.[8]

Less than a month later, an outbreak of highly pathogenic H7N2 was identified in a flock of chickens in Pocomoke City, Maryland. On Sunday, March 7, a total of 118,000 farm birds were culled, and another 210,000 birds on a second farm, under the same ownership, were destroyed the following day. Later that week, another 40,000 chickens from a third farm owned by the same farmer were also destroyed.[9]

The preceding chronology illustrates that avian influenza outbreaks have occurred in the U.S. with varying degrees of severity for many years. Taken in context, these incidents raise a very real concern about economic losses to the poultry industry. If H5N1 is detected in U.S. flocks, the financial consequences to the poultry sector could be dire. However, the nation and the economy have weathered HPAI outbreaks in the past; These outbreaks are nothing new. Keep that in mind—and don't panic—if and when the media starts hawking that H5N1 has arrived in this country.

One other critically important consideration needs to be kept in mind. Past experiences with H5N1 and other HPAI outbreaks have a striking similarity to the current bird flu hysteria: Reports of human deaths have been exceedingly rare.

HIGHLY PATHOGENIC AVIAN INFLUENZA (HPAI) OUTBREAKS[10]

Year	Country / Area	Domestic Bird Affected	Strain
1959	Scotland	Chicken	H5N1
1963	England	Turkey	H7N3
1966	Ontario (Canada)	Turkey	H5N9
1976	Victoria (Australia)	Chicken	H7N7
1979	Germany	Chicken	H7N7
1979	England	Turkey	H7N7
1983-1985	Pennsylvania (USA)*	Chicken, Turkey	H5N2
1983	Ireland	Turkey	H5N8
1985	Victoria (Australia)	Chicken	H7N7
1991	England	Turkey	H5N1
1992	Victoria (Australia)	Chicken	H7N3
1994	Queensland (Australia)	Chicken	H7N3
1994-1995	Mexico*	Chicken	H5N2
1994	Pakistan*	Chicken	H7N3
1997	New South Wales (Australia)	Chicken	H7N4
1997	Hong Kong (China)*	Chicken	H5N1
1997	Italy	Chicken	H5N2
1999-2000	Italy*	Turkey	H7N1
2002	Hong Kong (China)	Chicken	H5N1
2002	Chile	Chicken	H7N3
2003	Netherlands*	Chicken	H7N7

*Outbreaks with significant spread to numerous farms, resulting in great economic losses. Most other outbreaks involved little or no spread from the initially infected farms. Printed with permission from WHO.

Drifting and shifting: How viruses change

For symptoms to occur, a virus must undergo replication. Only when a virus bypasses through several layers of immune system protection can it proliferate and trigger the cascade of symptoms associated with the flu.

Viral replication is a complex task, and defects can occur during the process, resulting in offspring that are not exact copies of its parent. If a small alteration in the genetic makeup of an influenza virus is repeated, it is said to become a permanent change in the genes of the virus, creating a brand-new strain. Even though the new strain is related to the parent virus, the subtle differences make it "antigenically distinct," meaning that it seems like a brand-new virus to the immune system. This change, called an antigenic "drift," accounts for the differences in each year's influenza viruses. The CDC takes advantage of this drift, using it to justify the production of a new flu shot each season.

But major changes in the surface for antigens of viruses can also occur, leading to what is called an antigenic shift. Conditions favorable for the development of an antigenic shift have long been blamed on humans who live in close proximity to domestic poultry and pigs. For example, if the human influenza virus H3N2 infects a pig that is simultaneously harboring any one of the avian influenza viruses (say, H6N4 from a chicken), the two viruses have an opportunity to exchange genes. The new "recombinant" virus will contain genetic material from both parent viruses. This process—the blending of two different viruses—is called "reassortment." Mixing of surface antigens can lead to a new virus that the human immune system has had no previous exposure, sparking a global pandemic.

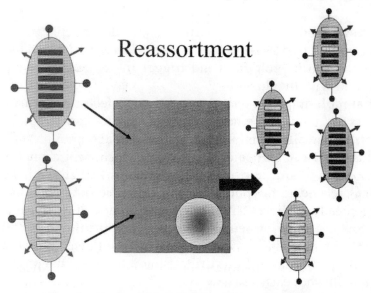

Diagram reproduced with permission from Dr. Vikram Misra, professor and head of the Department of Microbiology, Western College of Veterinary Medicine, University of Saskatchewan. (Slide #15 of presentation.)[11]

Reassortment and antigenic shifts are what scientists are worried about. They fear that a new "super influenza virus" could emerge and be particularly dangerous to humans, depending on which gene or genes are acquired during the swap. Antigenic shifts have been blamed for all three influenza pandemics. For example, it is thought that the reassortment of a human H2 antigen with the avian H3 antigen was the origin of the new H3N2 virus outbreak that caused the pandemic of 1968. And antigenic shift is the most widely held theory for the start of the 1918 influenza pandemic.[12]

Antigenic Shift

Monitoring the tendency of influenza viruses to undergo antigenic drifts and shifts has been the work of the World Health Organization (WHO) Global Influenza Program since its inception in 1947. Shifts occur annually and are the basis for adjusting the composition of each year's influenza vaccine. The current concern is that a major change in the (H) and/or (N) viral surface proteins will occur, igniting the next global pandemic.

A pandemic by definition is an outbreak of a disease occurring over a very wide area, crossing international boundaries and usually affecting a large number of people. It has been long held that the 1918 pandemic virus emerged through the combination of an influenza virus from a bird and an influenza virus from a pig combined, resulting in a new virus that massively infected humans. A variation of this concept is that the 1918 pandemic virus arose from the combination of a human H1N1 virus with a swine virus while both viruses were co-infecting a pig.[13] Either way, the long held assumption has been that the 1918 virus arose from the process of reassortment: Humans, birds, and pigs living close enough together that the viruses had the opportunity to swap genes.[14]

However, recent research has challenged the theory of reassortment, speculating that the 1918 virus didn't come from "gene swapping" after all, but started from a bird flu virus that "jumped species" and infected humans directly without an intermediary, meaning that antigenic shift wasn't involved after all. The new theory states that bird flu viruses can directly infect humans and lead to another pandemic.

Government scientists recently released what has been called the "definitive evidence" identifying the 1918 virus as a bird virus that "jumped species" and infected humans directly. The work involved the recreation of crushed viruses extracted from lung tissue of two soldiers and an Alaskan woman who died during the 1918 pandemic. The soldiers' tissue samples had been saved in an Army pathology warehouse, and the woman's remains had been preserved in a mass grave in the permanently frozen ground. "We now think that the 1918 virus was an entirely avian-like virus that adapted to humans," said Dr. Jeffery Taubenberger, researcher from the Armed Forces Institute of Pathology.[15] The report, a culmination of 10 years of work, was published in two respected journals, *Science* and *Nature*, in October 2005.

The publication date certainly seems timely. It legitimizes worries that bird flu can be transmitted directly to humans and plays into the hands of those who are spending billions of dollars to prepare for an outbreak of avian flu.

From my rotting body, flowers shall grow and
I am in them and that is eternity.
~Edvard Munch, Artist

Chapter 4: Perspective From Past Pandemics

Starting points:
- Three major influenza pandemics of the 21st century
- Lessons learned from past pandemics

The CDC and WHO continue to warn we that are overdue for the next pandemic. Forecasters are calling for the next global pandemic, similar to the Great Influenza Pandemic of 1918 in which tens of millions reportedly died from the flu. Three major pandemics have occurred in this past century. It is the pattern of these outbreaks that have the global authorities and the media concerned.[1]

Ten influenza pandemics, defined by clinical and epidemiological records, have occurred in the last 300 years. The serotypes of six outbreaks have been identified.

H2N2 (1889)	H2N2 (1957)
N3N8 (1900)	H3N2 (1968)
H1N1 (1918)	H1N1 (1977)

Spanish Flu (1918–1919)

The most highly discussed outbreak is the global influenza pandemic of 1918. It has been reported that more than 200 million people were ill due to the virus, but death estimates range from 30 to 100 million, an ever-changing and escalating number. Adjusting for today's population, the CDC estimates a similar pandemic would yield a modern death toll of 175 to 350 million. Called the Spanish flu, it gained its name from the press in politically neutral Spain, where some of the earliest printed reports of the flu's impact were not censored during World War I.

The pandemic reportedly began with a relatively mild "herald wave" in the spring of 1918. Many flu-like symptoms were recorded that spring: sore throat, headache, fever, and loss of appetite. Even though the geographic origin of the epidemic is still debated, the most widely accepted location is Fort Riley, an army camp located in Haskell County, Kansas.

On the morning of March 4, 1918, the company cook, Albert Gitchell, reported to duty with a temperature of 103°F (39.5°C). He was soon followed by Corporal Lee Drake and Sergeant Adolph Hurby. Within two days 522 men at the camp were sick. Throughout the summer, infections became increasingly more severe. By mid-August, three significant outbreaks had been reported that seemed to be completely unrelated because they occurred in such disparate locations: Brest, France; Boston, Massachusetts; and Freetown, Sierra Leone. Among U.S. military personnel, death rates reportedly ranged from 5 to 10 percent of those afflicted. While it is clear that those who were most ill were soldiers, the virus also spread throughout civilian populations. People without symptoms could be struck suddenly and rendered too feeble to walk within hours; Many would die the next day. A key symptom was the presence of cyanosis, a blue discoloration to the face due to rapid accumulation of fluid in the lungs. Severe cases often required hospitalization. Not surprisingly, even with the best available care of the day, nearly one-third of those infected reportedly died.[2]

The highest mortality rate occurred among those who developed a rapidly progressing pneumonia. Because penicillin was not discovered until 1928, many deaths were most likely due to secondary bacterial infections, and could have been preventable today. As pointed out in a letter published in the *Wall Street Journal* on November 1, 2005, by Dr. Edward H. Livingston, chairman of gastrointestinal and endocrine surgery at the University of Texas Southwestern School of Medicine, hospitalization at the turn of the century didn't have much to offer. Even the use of intravenous therapy, routine today, was virtually nonexistent in 1918. His astute comments included, "In 1918, care of the flu patient was limited to rest, providing aspirin, oxygen, and other supportive measures. The primary cause of death was pneumonia resulting from bacterial infection of lungs injured as a result of the flu. Lacking antibiotics, there was no effective way of treating the pneumonia."[3]

A unique feature of the 1918 influenza pandemic was the demographics of the people who were most likely to die. Normally, flu is only life-threatening to the very old, the very young and people with compromised immune systems. But in 1918, men between the ages of 20 and 40 were the most common victims; in fact, men were 35 percent more likely than women to die from flu.[4] This statistic is left unexplained in the history books, but perhaps, exposes a clue that requires further exploration. In addition to the lack of progressive care, the true mortality numbers are unknown. In 1999, the CDC claimed that 20 million died in the 1918 pandemic. In 2005, it claimed 50 million. The discrepancy is given a broad brush in the media, which reports the number of deaths ranged from 20 to 100 million. Certainly, many died, but the exaggerations accentuate the hype and conveniently ignore the societal and healthcare advances of the last 100 years. The early 1900s were characterized by a lack of medical technology, minimal means of communication, and no consistent household registration system. Pubic health departments had barely been conceived. Given all this, it is impossible for the global mortality figures and projected estimates to be accurate.

During a CDC press briefing teleconference on November 2, 2005, John Wellerman of *Bloomberg News* asked a direct question of the CDC panel: "I want to find out why the estimates of [anticipated] deaths from the pandemic have increased so much. I believe last year the studies said 200,000 people might be killed by pandemic. This iteration says 1.9 million."

The director of the National Vaccine Program, Dr. Bruce Gelling, fielded the question and responded, "We actually provide two estimates, and one of them is based on the 1957–1958 pandemic, which, in looking back over pandemics, was relatively mild.... We don't know what the H5N1 virus will do, we don't know what any virus will do, but we felt that it would be best suited *to have our preparations based on that worst case,* which is, in modern memory, 1918." (Emphasis added.)[5]

After the initial outbreaks in 1918, subsequent milder waves continued to occur over the next two years. Within months after its onset, the 1918 flu epidemic disappeared as rapidly as it began. Did the virus mutate? Did people who were exposed develop a natural immunity to the virus? Or did something in the environment change, making people less susceptible to the flu?

Asian Flu (1957–1958)

The new influenza virus, H2N2, was isolated in Singapore in February 1957 arriving in Hong Kong later that year. The new flu strain that had circulated throughout the southern hemisphere arrived in the U.S. during June 1957. Ultimately blamed for the deaths of nearly 70,000 Americans, the H2N2 virus is thought to have originated from the reassortment of genes from wild ducks. Notably different from the 1918 pandemic, the highest mortality rates occurred among the elderly. Worldwide, one million people reportedly died during the 1957 flu pandemic.

Hong Kong Flu (1968–1969)

When the novel subtype virus, H3N2, was first identified in Hong Kong on August 16, 1968, WHO rapidly issued a warning: Another worldwide outbreak was looming. It was predicted that the outbreak pattern would be similar to that seen in 1957, but this pandemic was different. Nearly everywhere, the clinical symptoms were mild and the mortality was low. The disease seemed to spread slowly rather than explosively. In some countries, absentee rates and increased deaths rates were slight or non-existent.

Canada, for example, experienced practically no deaths from the flu. In the U.K., deaths from influenza-like illness and pneumonia were actually *lower* than in the year preceding the new outbreak. A similar picture was seen in most of Europe, where flu symptoms were mild and excessive deaths were negligible. In striking contrast, the influenza outbreaks across the U.S. were the notable global exceptions. Nearly 34,000 deaths were attributed to the influenza, mostly in the elderly.[6]

Researchers suggest that the death rate may have been lower worldwide because the strain had a shift in the (H) antigen only—from H2 to H3—and the (N) antigen remained the same as the virus that was associated with the 1957 outbreak. People who had been exposed to that virus 10 years earlier had an intrinsic resistance, resulting in far fewer casualties. However convenient this explanation appears to be, it doesn't explain the skew toward the elderly. Most in that age group would also have been previously exposed to the 1957 viruses that supposedly made this pandemic less severe.

Summary of WHO "Lessons Learned" from Previous Pandemics

1. Pandemics behave as unpredictably as the viruses that cause them.
2. The severity of illness cannot be known in advance.
3. The pandemic may cause severe disease in young adults, a major determinant of overall impact.
4. The epidemiological potential of a virus tends to unfold in waves.
5. Viral surveillance by WHO laboratories is critically important.
6. Most pandemics have originated in parts of Asia where dense populations of humans live in close proximity to ducks and pigs.
7. **Quarantine and travel restrictions have shown little effect.** [Emphasis added.]
8. Delaying spread is desirable so that fewer people at a time will require healthcare.
9. **The impact of vaccines on a pandemic remains to be demonstrated.** [Emphasis added.]
10. Countries with domestic manufacturing capacity will be the first to receive vaccines.
11. The interval between successive outbreak waves is unpredictable.
12. In the best-case scenario, a pandemic will cause excess mortality only at the extremes of life and in persons with underlying chronic disease. These are the same groups at high risk during the influenza season.

Lessons from past pandemics

The WHO has created a 12-point list of "lessons learned" from previous pandemics. However, a critical view of the three historical global influenza outbreaks can lead to different lessons than those deduced by the WHO:[7]

1. Malnutrition played a role in the 1918 pandemic.

Whereas fit and healthy persons are resistant to infections under ordinary circumstances, wars, chemical exposures, and other natural disasters can lead to increased susceptibility. During wartime, malnutrition due to shortages of fresh food and an absence of clean water can lead to widespread immunocompromise. In 1985, the director of the National Institute of Allergy and Infectious Disease (NIAID), Dr. Anthony Fauci, declared that malnutrition was the most prevalent cause of immune deficiency diseases throughout the world in humans.[8] Malnutrition undoubtedly played a hefty role in the large number of deaths during the 1918 pandemic.

2. Two of the three pandemics were directly associated with wars.

Global outbreaks of influenza occurred around the time of American-involved wars: World War I and Vietnam. In fact, the WHO attributed the 1968 outbreak to the return of U.S. troops to California from Southeast Asia.[9] Poor hygiene, emotional stress, pre-deployment vaccines, and chemical exposure contributed to the weakening of immune systems and outbreak of influenza.

3. The general health of those who contracted influenza is unknown.

During the global outbreaks, the underlying health conditions of those who died are unknown. Influenza could have been blamed for deaths that were really caused by something else, such as congestive heart failure or bacterial pneumonia.

4. Healthcare technology has advanced, leading to increased chances of survival.

Dramatic advances in medicine, public sanitation, personal hygiene, and food preparation make it much less likely that a naturally occurring pandemic of global proportion will ever happen again.

5. Vaccination could have contributed to influenza deaths.

Before going to war in 1918, troops received the smallpox and yellow fever vaccinations and possibly several more. Worldwide smallpox vaccination had been ongoing since the late 1800s. The Salk polio vaccination campaign began in 1955; the Asian flu outbreak occurred shortly thereafter (1957). The young men who served in Vietnam—and those who served stateside—received many vaccines, including an experimental plague vaccine, before deployment and the start of the 1968 pandemic.[10]

The impact of mass vaccination on the troops and within the civilian population could have led to immune system disruption, increasing susceptibility to the effects of influenza viruses.

5. The present healthcare financing model makes the influenza vaccine unattractive

Within the global economics, the healthcare delivery structures of those who can afford it pay... today... would have been... claims for a product that none could ... be...commanding... high price ...

6. Regulatory uncertainty, has deterred leading to increased manufacturer shutdown.

... regulatory uncertainty, ... makes public health, scarcity of resources and low ... paces, make ... in every case, ... likely to disrupt the tendency of vaccine production will ever improve ...

8. Tactics that could have controlled attacks influenza deaths

... shown that in ... vaccine. ... however, the strategies ... ... conditions, and ... ... has been available, ... infection or ... have median ... the ... ... population... ... the ... ... the obligation ... and those with serious health conditions ... ... the ... an ... ... the serum from ... ... than ... ... the vaccine ... ... or more to the most vulnerable ... ... the impact of ... vaccine on ... ... an attack that ... ... any ... ... the ... influenza season, ... people share a lineage ... not the vaccine program ...

30

Power concedes nothing without a demand…. Find out just what
people will submit to and you have found out the exact amount of
injustice and wrong which will be imposed upon them….
~Frederick Douglass, Human Rights Activist

Chapter 5: Recent Fiascos: The Swine Flu and the Smallpox Scare

Starting points:
- The swine flu scare of 1976
- The smallpox scare of 2002
- Dispelling the smallpox myths

Since the 1970s, epidemiologists have observed that major antigenic shifts seem to occur in 11-year cycles, beginning with an outbreak of the flu in 1946–47. It has also been suggested that the strains "recycle" their surface antigens about every 50 years, long enough that most people who had experienced the flu and had developed an innate immunity to the virus within a population would have died.

The 11-year model appeared to apply, since there were exactly 11 years between the pandemics of 1946, 1957, and 1968. Also, historical comparisons showed that the 1957 disease was similar to the 1889 disease, and the 1968 disease was similar to that of 1900.[1]

However, the convenient construct of an 11-year cycle fell apart when no pandemic appeared in 1979, although many *thought* one was about to occur in 1976. That would-be pandemic became the fiasco called the swine flu.

Fort Dix: Where it began

Even though April 30, 1975, marked the end of the U.S. presence in Vietnam, young men across the country continued to sign up for the all-volunteer army. Just after the Christmas holiday in 1975, thousands of enthusiastic new army recruits reported to the barracks at Fort Dix, New Jersey, to begin basic training. However, by mid-January, many were complaining of flu-like symptoms; a few had even been hospitalized.

One recruit reported to his drill instructor that he felt tired and weak. Given the option to rest, he opted instead to participate in a five-mile training march on a cold February night. Twenty-four hours later, on February 6, 1975, the 19-year-old Pvt. David Lewis of Ashley Falls, Massachusetts, was dead. Word arrived the following week from the CDC laboratory that his death was caused by an influenza type A virus. Particularly worrisome was that four other samples taken from ill recruits at Fort Dix had also tested positive for influenza A virus—a type that had previously been detected only in pigs.

Alarms started to sound throughout the public health sector. If a pig virus had "jumped species" and directly infected a human, was this the start of another pandemic?

On February 20, 1976, the *New York Times* ran a story titled "U.S. Calls Flu Alert on Possible Return of Epidemic Virus." Experts said that there was "little danger of any 'wildfire' epidemic on the newly found virus," and that the flu cluster at Fort Dix may be nothing more than a "curiosity." However, what started as a possible fluke quickly ramped up to a national emergency.[2]

Within three weeks of Lewis' death, researchers and public health officials converged in Washington to persuade members of Congress to implement a costly new program involving the rapid development of a novel vaccine and to implement an expanded program of mass vaccination.

A nationwide campaign, launched with the urgency of a five-alarm fire, was started by the CDC in search of other persons who had been infected with the swine flu virus. In addition to a few earlier cases reported in Minnesota and Wisconsin, already known to the CDC, the investigation turned up isolated occurrences throughout Pennsylvania, Virginia, and Mississippi. Every case, except for one questionable instance in Virginia, involved human-to-pig contact.

By March 15, word reached President Ford by way of the CDC that the country was on the verge of a major influenza pandemic. Calling an urgent meeting with his top advisors including, among others, Richard Cheney and Donald Rumsfeld, the president was unanimously urged to begin preparing for a massive vaccination program. As a point of caution, Ford postponed his decision until he had the assurances of scientists on how to proceed. The following week, Ford met with a blue-ribbon panel of experts from the CDC and the National Institutes of Health (NIH), including renowned polio vaccine experts Drs. Jonas Salk and Albert Sabin. Hearing the consensus from his team that the massive program was not only necessary but also critically important, the president presented his case to the American people on March 24, 1976. During the nationally televised address, he announced the formation of the National Influenza Immunization Program and a plan for the mass vaccination of all Americans. At the same time, the president appealed to Congress for the funds to make it happen.

With unparalleled haste, Rep. Paul G. Rogers (D-FL), chairman on Health and the Environment, rushed bill HR 13012 through his subcommittee and sent it directly to the House floor on April 5. Even though most members of the House had neither seen nor read the legislation, the bill passed that same day by a vote of 354–12. With only minor modifications, the Senate approved the appropriations for the bill, 61–7, a mere four days later.[3]

Now that the money was in place for a vaccination program— funded by taxpayers—all that was needed was a vaccine.

Recent painful memories for pharma

Almost immediately, liability protection emerged as an issue for the vaccine makers. Vaccine injury lawsuits were a recent memory in the minds of the insurance underwriters, having weathered the storms of litigation with Cutter Laboratories during the implementation of the polio vaccine program. In 1955, Cutter was one of several pharmaceutical companies licensed to produce Salk's killed-virus polio vaccine. Through a series of errors, thousands of vaccine lots containing live virus had been released to the general public, causing polio and severe illness in more than 40,000 children; 200 became permanently paralyzed and 10 died.

The ensuing, 28-day jury trial took place in Oakland's Alameda County Superior Court. In the end, the jury found that Cutter was not negligent in the production of the vaccine, but nonetheless awarded one victim $147,300. The court reasoned Cutter had met production standards of the day, but was liable for marketing a vaccine it claimed was safe when clearly it was not. The verdict, upheld on appeal, opened the door for more lawsuits against makers of vaccines and drove Cutter out of the vaccine business.[4]

The damage award was not monumental, even by 1955 standards, but the problems and risks associated with vaccines were enough to get the attention of the manufacturers' insurance companies. Refusing to issue insurance coverage that would protect the drug companies from lawsuits arising from side effects and complications of vaccines became the new rule. If it happened with the polio vaccine, it could certainly happen with other vaccines including the new, fast-tracked swine flu vaccine.

Once Congress announced it was willing to fund the swine flu program, the insurance companies made their positions known. On April 8, 1976, the Federal Insurance Company advised Merck that all liability, indemnity, and defense costs associated with claims arising from the swine flu vaccine would not be covered by its insurance plan. Within days, the other three vaccine manufacturers —Merrell, Parke-Davis and Wyeth—received similar notices. At about that same time, T. Lawrence Jones, president of the American Insurance Association, had a meeting with government officials letting them know that the insurance industry had no plans to insure any of the manufacturers for swine flu vaccine.

The pressure was on from all sides to get government money into the game. If the swine flu program was going to get off the ground, the federal government would have to put up the money—more tax dollars—to protect a private industry. The government would need to assume liability for any and all problems that could arise in persons who would receive the vaccine. Concerns were raised in Congress resulting in heated hearings, with some legislators arguing that passing protective legislation would lead to careless manufacturing on the part of the drug companies. Others argued that without the vaccine a raging epidemic could occur and production must continue at all costs.

In the heat of the debate, a strange outbreak was reported that shifted public opinion and secured all the benefits sought by the drug companies and their insurance underwriters. In early July 1976, an unusually deadly respiratory infection was occurring among guests attending a bicentennial celebration at the Bellevue-Stratford Hotel in Philadelphia. Within two days after the start of the annual American Legion Convention, one veteran after another became ill. Ultimately, 221 were stricken and 34 eventually died.

Fearing the worst, pandemonium broke out. Even though the disease did not clinically resemble influenza, Secretary of Health, Education, and Welfare (HEW) David Mathews suggested there was a "possibility" that the swine flu virus was causing the reported illnesses. Congress was forced by the press and a panicked public to halt the debates and take action. By August 12, President Ford had signed the National Swine Flu Immunization Program and Tort Claim Bill of 1976 into law.[5] With the funding in place for both the manufacture of the vaccine and for guaranteed liability protection, manufacturers had a green light to proceed with the development of the vaccine. A national program was launched with the intent of vaccinating every man, woman, and child in America with the swine flu vaccine.

It wasn't until six months later, on January 18, 1977, that the causative agent for Legionnaire's Disease—a bacterium—was discovered and ulimately named Legionella. Analysis revealed that the source of the organism was the hotel's water tower that circulated through its air conditioning system. Since that time, water-pumped air conditioning systems in the Bellevue-Stratford have been changed, and federal agencies have tightened regulations for public buildings that still have cooling towers as part of their air conditioning systems.

A Gallup Poll conducted in late August 1976 showed that 93 percent of Americans were aware of the immunization program, but only 52 percent intended to get the shot. A bigger push was needed to ensure the success of the lofty goals of a nationwide vaccination program. Based on the results of that August poll, an unprecedented national media campaign was launched to fully convince the wary public to participate. The government's unwavering message, sent out through every form of media, was that the vaccine was both "safe and necessary."

But not everyone was convinced, and the campaign had a few outspoken opponents.

Dr. Russell Alexander of the Public Health School at the University of Washington had emerged as the principal voice of reason, calling for further evidence before proceeding. His general view was that "you should be conservative about putting foreign material into the human body. That's always true…especially when you are talking about 200 million bodies. The need should be estimated conservatively. If you don't need to give it, don't."[6]

His views were strongly supported by the director of the New Jersey Public Health Laboratories, Dr. Martin Goldfield, who had first identified the virus at Fort Dix as a swine virus. He challenged the decision—made primarily by politicians—to mass vaccinate the general public. Ignoring the bureaucratic hierarchy, Goldfield fiercely expressed his opposition at CDC meetings, although he was repeatedly ignored. Out of frustration and serious concern for the public, he released his opinions to the rapacious press. A transcript of his interview on "The CBS Evening News" clearly documented Goldfield's position: "There are as many dangers to going ahead with immunizing the population as there are withholding. We can soberly estimate that approximately 15 percent of the entire population will suffer a disabling reaction [from the vaccine]."[7] This was not what the administration or public health stalwarts wanted the people to hear. Goldfield was relieved of his duties in 1977, suggesting that his outspoken opposition to mass vaccination may have cost him his job.

Another outspoken opponent, FDA Virus Bureau Director Dr. Anthony Morris (formerly of HEW), announced early on that a swine influenza vaccine could not be made because there had never been any cases of swine flu in humans to test its effectiveness. Dr. Morris warned his superiors in the federal government that the vaccine would be "dangerous and most likely ineffective," but they had no interest in his admonishments. Bypassing his superiors, he too went directly to the media warning the public that the vaccine was going to be unsafe and that an epidemic was unlikely to occur. As a result, he was fired from his position at the FDA, his experimental animals were destroyed, the publication of his findings was blocked, and the vaccine program moved forward unopposed.[8]

With the massive political buildup and momentum of the media pushing the program, cautious minds could not prevail. Public health officials from coast to coast felt they had an opportunity to do in 1976 what had not been done during the influenza outbreaks in 1957 or 1968. Most importantly, they could accomplish their goals using federal funds, with Congress assuming the liability and the president taking ultimate responsibility.

On October 1, 1976, the national vaccination campaign began, with the first shot given at the State Fair in Indianapolis, Indiana. Thousands of doctors, nurses, and paramedics across the country volunteered to give shots at medical centers, schools, and firehouses. Between the program's inception and its demise a few weeks later, approximately 40 million Americans—one-third of the adult population of the United States—were vaccinated. This made the swine flu campaign the largest vaccination program ever undertaken in U.S. history.

Almost as quickly as the program began, however, reports of casualties started to pour in. Three elderly Pittsburgh citizens who had been vaccinated at the same clinic died within several days of receiving the shot. Officials from the CDC were sent to investigate the deaths. Concluding that there was "no evidence to suggest" that the deaths were caused by the vaccine, the program was encouraged to continue.

Reports of deaths continued, and within two weeks of the launch of the program, 33 persons who had been injected with the vaccine had died. More foreboding were the dozens of reports of Guillain-

Barré syndrome (GBS), an inflammatory disorder of the peripheral nerves (those outside the brain and spinal cord). Called an ascending paralysis, GBS starts in the legs and moves up the body, quickly involving the muscles that aid in breathing, including the diaphragm, resulting in respiratory failure. Maximal muscle weakness typically occurs two weeks after the onset of GBS, and treatment often involves long-term, intensive care hospitalization, with most patients needing the assistance of a respirator.[9]

Despite widespread reports of death and paralysis, the publicity barrage continued, culminating on October 14, 1976, with the appearance of President Ford and his family receiving flu shots on national television, and encouraging all those who had not yet received the vaccine to do so as soon as possible.

But dissent was growing louder by the week, and the facts could not be ignored. The CDC's epidemiologists were clearly stating that there was no evidence of human-to-human transmission of the swine flu virus and that no further cases of the swine flu virus had occurred in humans. Nationwide, doctors were having second thoughts about administering the vaccine, and patients were mostly refusing it.

A mere six weeks after his dramatic vaccination and appeal to the general public, the president once again appeared on national TV, this time to concur with the CDC's decision to suspend the program –while defending the original decision to vaccinate the entire country to protect its citizens against swine flu. When the CDC issued a press release on December 14 stating that cases of GBS had been reported in ten states, enough was enough. The program was officially suspended.[10]

According to a report in *Newsweek* posted July 18, 1977, claims totaling more than $1.3 billion were filed by the 532 people who contracted GBS after vaccination. While many recovered in the ensuing months, 32 died and up to 10 percent remained paralyzed to varying degrees for

> GBS is believed to be an autoimmune response to a component within the swine flu vaccine; It can also be triggered by the seasonal influenza vaccine. An estimated 40 cases of GBS related to influenza vaccination occur in the U.S. annually.

the rest of their lives.

Because the drug companies had been protected by The Swine Flu Act, claims for compensation had to be filed with the federal government. The new secretary of HEW, Joseph A. Califano, Jr., responded to the difficulties experienced when the aftermath of the program erupted with litigation. He declared that, with respect to those alleging GBS, the policy of the government was "to provide compensation to all who contracted GBS from the swine flu vaccine without having to prove negligence." Instead, claimants needed to show only that they had, in fact, developed Guillain-Barré as a result of a swine flu vaccine and had suffered damages as a result of that condition. The secretary gave two reasons for this policy:

> "First, the informed consent form did not adequately warn individuals that there was a one in 100,000 risk that a person receiving the flu shot could contract Guillain-Barré and that one in every two million would die from the condition.... Second, in the swine flu program, the federal government, in an unprecedented effort, actively urged millions of Americans to get flu vaccinations and funded the nationwide campaign. Thus we have decided to provide just compensation for those who contracted Guillain-Barré as a result of the swine flu program rather than force many individuals to prove government negligence in protracted proceedings."[11]

Although Califano's statement, affirmed and upheld by the Tenth Circuit Court, appears to be a straightforward way to collect damages from the government, it took many years before the victims received their settlements.[12]

Skeptics say that the Ford administration, beleaguered by a stagnant economy and abashed by the Nixon pardon, was desperate for a rallying point. The swine flu crisis provided just what was needed. But whatever the motivations, less than 30 percent of the targeted number bothered to get vaccinated. Thirty years later, public policy experts remain divided on the appropriateness of Ford's action. In 1999, a belated postscript in *Time Magazine* ranked the swine flu program 85th on its list of the "100 Worst Ideas of the Century."[13]

And what came of the killer epidemic? It never emerged.

It is thought that the total number of cases attributed to swine flu was six, and perhaps it was really just one. With all the money spent and the many lives ruined, no outbreaks occurred following the initial few cases at Fort Dix.

A question comes to mind regarding the swine flu that has not previously been asked: Could the recruits at Fort Dix have been exposed to something, either intentionally or unintentionally, that led to an outbreak of the virus? During the height of the swine flu concern, antibody testing suggested that as many as 500 asymptomatic recruits had been exposed to the swine flu virus. None of the civilians or pigs on any of the farms in the surrounding area tested positive for the specific swine flu viral type seen in the recruits, and the WHO never detected any signs of the virus internationally. In addition, the swine flu virus was detected only at Fort Dix and no other military bases.

Could there have been a unique exposure to those arriving at Fort Dix? More likely than not, we will never know.[14]

Smallpox: Another type of scare; the same type of hype

Fast-forward 20 years.

The nation was starting to contemplate the possibility of an act of bioterrorism occurring on U.S. soil. Concerns were being raised in the public health sector about how to protect the country in the event of an attack with a biological weapon. As early as 1999, 21 representatives from major medical and research centers, government, the military, public health, and emergency management institutions and agencies met to develop a plan to protect the civilian population in the event of a terrorist attack.[15]

And then, the events of 9-11 occurred.

The aftermath of those events included the discovery of anthrax spores in Congressional quarters. Iraqi President Saddam Hussein was thought to be harboring massive canisters of anthrax and smallpox and the prevailing sentiment was that he could be planning an immediate attack. Something needed to be done to prepare for the worst.

Just as in the discovery of the lone swine flu case, government officials were off and running without a single case. The flurry of activity was based only on a *presumption.*

Nevertheless, the CDC was one step ahead of the game this time. Serendipitously, and somewhat eerily, the new recommendations for using the smallpox vaccine had been issued in June 2001, an update of a policy that had not been reviewed for more than 10 years.[16] With the resolutions in place, the government began to throw billions of dollars toward its customary public health solution–massive vaccination.

Contrasting sharply with the swine flu campaign, post 9-11 planning went beyond bureaucratic meetings and opening the government's coffers. The CDC held unprecedented town meetings in select locations across the country to elicit feedback from local public health officials and concerned citizens about the possibility of mandatory mass vaccination with the smallpox vaccine. (I was able to participate in two of the CDC town meetings, one in St. Louis and one in Atlanta.) Simultaneous with the town meetings, the media was ramping up, making dire predictions of massive death rates from the scourge of smallpox. The specter of mandatory vaccination erupted across the front page of newspapers and rode the radio airwaves. Experts on the subject were guests on television talk shows from Oprah to O'Reilly.

In the midst of the drama, factual discrepancies about smallpox began to appear. What was being propagated by the government and parroted by the media as "generally accepted facts" about smallpox simply weren't the real facts at all. Just as refuting those myths was important to calming the public's fears about smallpox, understanding that the same hyperbole is being used to fan the flames of fear about bird flu will serve to quell public fears now.

Myth #1: Smallpox is highly contagious.

Fact #1: No, it is not.

During the town meeting in St. Louis on June 8, 2002, Dr. Joel Kuritsky, Director of the National Immunization Program and the Early Smallpox Response and Planning Task Force at the CDC, stated, "Smallpox has a slow transmission and is not highly contagious." That is a direct contradiction to nearly everything that was being said, and being written, about smallpox.

Correspondingly, bird flu is not highly contagious. There has been no sustained person-to-person transmission, and humans seem to be highly resistant to developing problems thought to be associated with the H5N1 virus. The September 29, 2005, issue of the *New England Journal of Medicine* reported the following:

> "The relatively low frequencies of influenza A(H5N1) illness in humans, despite widespread exposure to infected poultry, indicate that the **species barrier to acquisition of this avian virus is substantial.** [Emphasis added.] Clusters of cases in family members may be caused by common exposures, although the genetic factors that may affect a host's susceptibility to disease warrant study."[17]

In plain language, this means that even with constant exposure to the virus, most persons are highly resistant to H5N1 and do not develop symptoms of the flu. Keep in mind that H5N1 has been around for many years. It hasn't "jumped species" so far; It is highly unlikely it will do so at any time in the future.

Myth #2: Smallpox is easily spread by casual contact with an infected person.

Fact #2: No, it is not.

Smallpox will not rapidly disseminate throughout the community. "The infection is spread by droplet contamination, coughing or sneezing is not generally part of the infection. Smallpox will **not** spread like wildfire," said Dr. Walter A. Orenstein, director of the CDC's National Immunization Program (NIP), at the town meeting in Atlanta on June 20, 2002.

CDC officials also set the record straight about the spread of smallpox. At the Atlanta town meeting, Dr. Kuritsky stated, "Given the slow transmission rate and that people need to be in close contact *for nearly a week* to spread the infection, the scenario in which a terrorist could infect himself with smallpox and contaminate an entire city by walking through the streets touching people *is purely fiction.*" [Emphasis added.] He went on to describe that 37 percent of smallpox cases in Africa and India had a transmission of only one generation, meaning that if a second person contracted smallpox, he did not pass it onto a third person. This explanation from the heads of the CDC directly contradicts models reported in the news that predicted an exponential spread to millions.

Similar to the media myth of rapid smallpox spread, there is no meaningful person-to-person transmission with bird flu. In one of the few cases in which an entire family in Thailand became infected (called a "cluster"), nine of those who were ill had had a clear history of direct contact with poultry. Because they were from the same household, they could have had a clustered exposure to an environmental contaminant. Even though several in this family were ill, there was no definitive evidence of human-to-human transmission.[18]

Further substantiating the lack of person-to-person transmission, there has been essentially no transmission of the virus from patients to healthcare workers in hospital settings, even when appropriate isolation measures were not used.[19] In fact, there has been only one confirmed case of person-to-person transmission–between an adult woman and her aunt during unprotected exposure to the critically ill patient.[20] Without person-to-person transmission there can be no pandemic. As with smallpox, the bird flu pandemic hype may turn out to be nothing more than purely fiction.

Myth #3: The death rate from smallpox is 30 percent.

Fact #3: The death rate from smallpox was 4.2 to 15 percent.[21]

Nearly every newspaper, magazine article, and television report before and after 2002 has quoted the CDC-generated statistic of a 30 percent death rate from smallpox. However, Dr. Tom Mack, retired from the University of Southern California (USC) and the CDC, reported at the Atlanta town meeting that the 30 percent fatality rate came from skewed data. Mack claimed to have seen more than 120 smallpox outbreaks in Pakistan during his career at the CDC in the 1970s. His observation was that villages would have an outbreak every five to ten years, *regardless of vaccination rate,* and the outbreak could always be predicted by living conditions and social arrangements. Many cases never came to the attention of the local authorities because they were so mild, the person did not seek medical attention.

Mack stated that even with poor medical care, the case fatality rate in adults was "much lower than is generally advertised" and was really much closer to 10 or 15 percent. His perception was that the statistics were "loaded with children that had a much higher fatality," skewing the death rate much higher, since children are not candidates for the vaccine. He revealed his opinion that even without mass vaccination, "smallpox would have died out anyway. It just would have taken longer." The information in quotation marks was taken verbatim from the transcript of the CDC town meeting held in Atlanta on June 19 and 20, 2002. This document, which I have in my possession, is no longer available online. The CDC has replaced the transcript of the town meeting with a summary.

Similarly, the actual death rate from bird flu, reported by the media to be nearly 50 percent, is completely unknown. Only the deaths of very ill persons who died in hospitals and had a positive test for H5N1 have been reported. Given how many people in Southeast Asia and across the globe live with and handle poultry, there is a high probability that large numbers of them have had uneventful contact with the H5N1 virus. Farmers in Southeast Asia literally sleep with their birds, and there has been no transmission from birds-to-humans.[22]

Hundreds, perhaps thousands, of individuals with H5N1 influenza have not been sick enough to require medical care, as confirmed by Dick Thompson, spokesperson for the WHO. In an interview with *CIDRAP News* in March 2005, Thompson stated, "The obvious assumption is that others are infected and either not getting sick, or not getting sick enough to seek treatment at a hospital. Factoring those patients into the death rate [makes it] impossible to determine, because the denominator is unknown."[23]

Dr. John Allen Paulos, professor of mathematics at Temple University, concurred with Thompson's observation. Paulos asserted that the reported death rate, based only on cases of severely ill persons, is an "almost textbook case" of sample bias. He explained that asymptomatic people, and those who have recovered uneventfully, aren't part of the mortality rate calculations. As a consequence, the numbers are skewed substantially upward.[24] Therefore, the reported fatality rate of close to 50 percent— like the smallpox 30 percent fatality rate—is being promoted for the sole purpose of frightening the public into accepting massive government regulations and submitting to vaccination.

Myth #4: There is no treatment for smallpox.

Fact #4: There are no pharmaceutical drugs for the treatment for smallpox.

Throughout history, smallpox infections occurred in varying degrees of severity. The most common form, called "ordinary discrete smallpox," occurred in more than 40 percent of cases. The outbreak manifested as a small scattering of pustules distributed across the body. The person was marginally ill and required minimal medical care. For mild cases, adequate hydration and fever control for comfort, and maintaining a temperature below 102°F (38.8°C), was all that was necessary. Keeping the skin clean to prevent bacterial infections was also important.

The 1927 *Textbook of Medicine* recommended applying gauze soaked in carbolic acid to "decrease itching and prevent extensive scarring." Carbolic acid was used acutely in the past for burns that tend to ulcerate and other skin conditions that cause burning or prickling pain. It was used routinely for smallpox.

Myth #5: The vaccine will prevent infection.

Fact #5: It will not.

Most people believe that vaccines prevent them from contracting a disease—a 200-year-old premise that is simply not true. Further, it is assumed that the presence of a vaccine-induced antibody will prevent an infection—another unproven assumption. The measurement of an amount of antibody in the blood is called a titer. Titers have not been proven to correlate with protection.[25] Many written reports and clinical observations have verified that fully vaccinated persons with adequate levels of "protective antibodies" can contract the illness for which they have been vaccinated.

Moreover, a negative can't be proven. For example, if a person receives a vaccine and does not become ill, is it due to the "protection" of the vaccine? Perhaps the person wasn't exposed to the microbe. Or, perhaps the person's immune system was resilient due to a good diet, adequate hygiene, etc. Proof that the vaccine prevents infection is virtually impossible.

Even the CDC admits that the smallpox vaccine did not prevent infection. Dr. Harold Margolis, senior advisor to the director of the CDC's Smallpox Planning and Response task force, stated at the St. Louis town meeting that "the vaccine decreased the death rate among those vaccinated by 'modifying the disease,' *not by preventing infection.*" [Emphasis added.] That means, if individuals had been vaccinated, they had a milder case of the disease…but they still got the disease.

Likewise, a person can get the flu shot and still get the flu. Even with the flu shot, adults can get one to three episodes, and children can get three to six episodes of influenza-like illness each year. An "influenza-like illness" is a respiratory infection characterized by fever, fatigue, cough, and other symptoms that are identical to the flu but not caused by an influenza virus. The CDC admits that the flu shot will not prevent influenza-like illnesses, therefore, "many persons who get the flu shot will still get the flu."[26] Keep this in mind when the push for the bird flu vaccine begins.

Another government-funded vaccine

In spite of the candid comments about smallpox that public health officials made at government-sponsored town meetings in 2002, stories of "what would happen in the event of an outbreak" continued to appear in the mainstream media. In addition, billions of dollars were poured into emergency planning. On May 5, 2003, Director of HHS Tommy Thompson announced the release of $100 million to "strengthen the public health infrastructure in preparation for a bioterrorism event." The funds, immediately available, were in addition to the $1.1 billion set aside in fiscal year 2002 for preparations at the state level and the $1.4 billion already allocated in 2003 for preparations at the national level. This increased the total expenditures in 2003 for bioterrorism preparedness, including research into potential disease agents, treatments, and vaccines, to $3.5 billion—up substantially from funds allocated in 2002.[27]

The media hype didn't end when the immediate smallpox concern subsided. In fact, as recently as January 2005, a made-for-television movie aired on the FX channel that was designed to show what could happen to a community if smallpox arrived in its town. "Smallpox" was produced in documentary style, creating a fictionalized "look back" to the year 2002 when a smallpox outbreak killed 60 million people. The tag line for the movie was "It's all true. It just hasn't happened yet."

When President Carter was sworn into office in 1977, the backwash of the swine flu program was still in full swing at the beginning of his term in office. His administration asked Drs.

Bioterrorism bills passed and funded with many billions of tax dollars since September 2001:

- U.S. PATRIOT Act, HR 3162, signed October 26, 2001
- Homeland Security Act, HR 5005, signed November 19, 2002
- Domestic Security Enhancement Act, signed December 23, 2003
- Project BioShield, S.15, signed July 21, 2004

Harvey Feinberg, who would become the 1982 president of the Institute of Medicine (IOM), and political historian, Richard Neustadt, to review the swine influenza program, focusing specifically on the decision-making processes. Their conclusions, compiled in the book *The Epidemic That Never Was* (1982), revealed significant flaws that led to crucial errors in decision-making during the swine flu program. The flaws included the following:

1. Overconfidence by specialists in theories that came from meager evidence.
2. Convictions that were fueled by preexisting personal agendas.
3. Zeal by health professionals at the CDC and NIH to pressure their lay superiors in government positions to "do the right thing."
4. Premature commitment to decisions without enough information.
5. Failure to address uncertainties in a way that allowed for reconsideration.
6. Insufficient questioning of scientific logic.
7. Insufficient questioning of the implementation program.
8. Insensitivity to media relations and to the long-term credibility of government institutions: CDC, NIH, and Congress.[28]

Feinberg and Neustadt were quick to observe that new influenza strains can occur in clusters, causing small outbreaks of human disease without becoming widespread. This is a lesson that current officials should be paying attention to as well.

The occurrences within the swine flu plan of 1976 and the smallpox plan of 2002 seem uncannily similar to the bird flu plan of 2005–6. The debatable point is whether the lessons from the past have not been learned, or whether the swine flu program has been used as a prototype for each successive financial grab by the pharmaceutical industry and political grab by controlling politicians.

After the initial media blitz and ensuing public panic about the potential bird flu pandemic, Americans have tended to fall back into their generally apathetic state. Recent events in politics have made the majority skeptical of government-backed fear messages, especially when they start out with zealous fanfare and nothing happens. Authorities need to do something to keep everyone psychologically concerned about about the possibility of the "death angel" sweeping round the globe while the vaccine is being developed and government programs are being solidified.

But the same messages are falling on deaf ears, and astute observers are seeing through the charade. An obvious example of the government's attempt to keep the fear going was the made-for-TV movie, "Fatal Contact: Bird Flu in America," broadcast on May 9, 2006. The movie aired on ABC during the May Sweeps in a morbid attempt to increase the network's ratings. In the television industry, the sweeps are when networks vie for the largest number of viewers so they can demand the highest rates for their ads over the upcoming months.

The promos portray the worst-case-scenario of a 1918-style, global pandemic. The previews show dead bodies so numerous that dump trucks were needed to haul them to funeral pyres. Barbed wire fences were used to quarantine entire neighborhoods. Anticipating that the movie would be very disturbing to viewers, officials prepared for the worst. The Pittsburgh Tribune Review reported that 15 phone lines in the studios at WTAE-TV were staffed by public health officials, infectious disease experts, mental health professionals and first responders armed with the "latest, most accurate information about the bird flu threat." People who were especially upset by the movie or concerned about the potential bird flu pandemic were to be referred to CONTACT Pittsburgh, the region's 24-hour crisis and suicide hotline.[29] As it turned out, the movie was an overwhelming flop. The ratings were dismal and less than five percent of the viewing audience actually watched the the poorly made docudrama.

The government is running out of time to find ways to keep us tuned into the potential seriousness of the pandemic. A plan was developed by experts in August 2005. Officials need to pull out that playbook and rework their plan.

50

We cannot banish dangers, but we can banish fears.
We must not demean life by standing in awe of death.
~David Sarnoff, Radio and Television Pioneer

Chapter 6: The New Playbook Arrives

Starting points:
- A review of the CDC's "Seven Step recipe" for media control
- SARS, the warm-up dance
- Keeping the heat on the hype: Enter the new ten-step plan
- Government crying wolf

The ho-hum attitude people are having about the overly hyped bird flu is the same attitude exhibited in the aftermath of the swine flu and smallpox programs. In fact, it's the same attitude more and more people are having toward the annual flu shot campaign—the frenzied reports have lost their effect and people have lost interest. Predictably, public health officials don't like it one bit.

Every winter it is reported that millions of people around the world get the flu. Co-workers and classmates are home for about a week, sick and miserable. A few—mostly the elderly and infirm—die. We're told the annual death toll exceeds 36,000 in the U.S. and a few hundred thousand around the globe. However, these numbers leave gaping holes in the government's credibility because medical authorities don't separate those who actually died of influenza from those who died of an "influenza-like illness" and complications such as pneumonia.

To ensure that everyone is appropriately conditioned to get a flu shot in the fall, the CDC developed a media plan, referred to as a "Seven Step Recipe for Generating Interest in, and Demand for, Flu (or Any Other) Vaccination," engineered to guarantee the economic success of each season's flu vaccine production line.[1]

The program is designed to methodically manipulate the general public through the use of major media (especially newswires and television) into believing that the influenza vaccine is absolutely necessary for the avoidance of the flu. The meticulously scheduled, mostly fear-based messages are aimed at convincing unsuspecting members of the public that the flu shot is necessary and they should be demanding it. By announcing the locations of flu shot clinics throughout a community, the local six o'clock news is even an accomplice, giving millions of dollars of free advertising to vaccine manufacturers.

Normally, the flu season is little more than a nuisance. Even major controversies like vaccine shortages and a contaminated vaccine supply that cut the number of doses by 50 percent barely made a blip on the proverbial radar screen for most people. For a few weeks in the fall of 2004, the media hyped the shortages and showed images of people standing in line for hours to be vaccinated. But by January so few had gotten flu shots that vaccine gluts led to the abandonment of rationing, and the authorities began once again to urge everyone to get in line.

Every fall, the usual "recipe" starts all over again in an attempt to ramp up the push for the annual flu vaccine. "Make a plan, then work the plan," comes to mind. But the same old plan has worn thin. The general public has come to understand that the flu isn't a catastrophic illness. The casual attitude most people have about the flu vaccine is the same attitude many are showing toward the frenzied reports of the impending bird flu—after an initial response, few are paying much attention. The government is finding it increasingly difficult to whip up fear about the avian flu, no matter how many articles or news reports of "catastrophic concern" are published.

But forecasting a possible disaster and being correct are two very different things. Governments and businesses worldwide felt the crushing economic consequences of the "epidemic hype" created in 2003 when officials erroneously predicted that the SARS outbreak was the start of the next global pandemic.

This is a summary of the presentation by Glen Nowak, PhD. His "Seven Step recipe," released for the 2004–5 influenza season, leaves little doubt how intensively the media is used to drive demand for the flu shot.

Step 1: Start discussing the flu at the beginning of the "immunization season."

Step 2: Media outlets are to make pronouncements that the "new strain" is anticipated to cause "severe illness and/or serious outcomes."

Step 3: Media is to invite local and national medical experts and public health authorities on as guests to "state concern and voice alarm (by predicting dire outcomes) and urge influenza vaccination."

Step 4: Reports by experts will be used to "frame the flu season in terms [that will] motivate behavior." Recommended language to be used includes "very severe," "more severe than last or past years," and, "deadly." Phrases should include "this could be the worst flu season ever," "the flu kills 36,000 people per year," and, "the flu shot is the best way to prevent the flu."

Step 5: The media is urged to report that influenza is causing "severe illness" and is "affecting lots of people." The intent is to "foster the perception" that the flu is serious without the vaccine.

Step 6: The media is given explicit instructions: Use pictures of people getting shots and find families who are willing to tell their story about the flu. The intent is **first to motivate, later to reinforce** the necessity of getting the flu shot.

Step 7: To drive the message home, television anchors are to make references to pandemic influenza and continually reinforce the importance of vaccination.

SARS: The warm-up dance

The first reported case of the "mysterious flu" was reported in South China in November 2002. Naming it SARS (Severe Acute Respiratory Syndrome), the WHO issued its first global alerts in early March 2003. Teams of experts were sent to investigate the outbreak. The hysteria grew quickly and within weeks the Hong Kong Department of Health issued an unprecedented quarantine order–keeping residents inside their homes. Shortly thereafter, Mainland China followed suit, closing public schools, cinemas, and libraries in an attempt to stop the spread of the virus.

Scientists went into high gear to determine the cause of SARS, and on April 16, 2003, the WHO announced that the infectant was discovered. It was a member of the coronavirus family, "never previously seen in humans." As more cases began to be reported in Toronto, Canadian health officials warned residents to quarantine themselves, wear masks, and in some cases, just stay home.

Over the six months of the "epidemic," 8,049 people had tested positive for the virus. The vast majority of cases occurred in China, Hong Kong, and Taiwan (7,248) with 774 deaths, or close to 10 percent of known cases. But since the total number of cases represented only those ill enough to seek medical help, the actual death rate is unknown and may have been far less.[2]

As for economic impact, even in Canada–where fewer people were affected (251) and even fewer (43) died–the Canadian Tourism Board estimated that the SARS scare cost the nation's economy $419 million. The Ontario health minister reported that the cost to the province's healthcare system, including money spent to develop special clinics and stock them with supplies to protect healthcare workers, was nearly $763 million.

SARS also had a significant, adverse effect on global travel, particularly the airline industry. Flights to Asia and the Pacific Rim decreased by 45 percent, and the number of flights between Hong Kong and the United States fell 69 percent.[3] Singapore Airlines, the world's second-largest airline by market value after U.S. budget carrier Southwest Airlines, lost $6 million *each day* during April and May when SARS choked off intra- and inter-Asian travel.[4]

Other less obvious industries throughout the region that suffered during the outbreak were retail sales, hotels, and restaurants. Additional losses resulted from workplace absenteeism. The WHO estimates that the economic consequences of SARS totaled more than $30 billion worldwide.[5] Undeniably, there is a genuine downside to issuing warnings that turn out to be unnecessary hype.

Unfortunately, avian influenza has inflicted similar economic consequences. Since the beginning of 2004, more than 200 million domestic birds have been killed in more than 10 countries, even if they were not known to be infected by the virus. The cost to various local economies is estimated to be in the tens of millions of dollars. And based on information being pumped out through every possible medium on a daily basis, the bird flu pandemic is still predicted to cause the "Next Great Depression" and "the end of life as we know it."[6]

Keeping the heat on the hype

But if the apocalypse is coming, only a few seem overly concerned. People seem to be mostly ignoring the gloomy scenarios being portrayed by the CDC and the WHO. Officials need to somehow capture the attention of the public, motivate participation in preparedness planning, and at the same time, maintain credibility.

Enter risk communication.

The field of risk communication is relatively new. Dating from the early 1980s, it evolved from several different fields of study: health education, public relations, psychology, risk perception, and risk assessment. Risk communication figured prominently in the CDC's commissioning of a new recipe, crafted by Princeton-based risk communication experts Peter M. Sandman, PhD and his wife, Jody Lanard, MD. Published in *Perspectives in Health,* their plan is based on the following three principles of risk communication:

- Precaution advocacy ("Watch out!"): How to alert people to serious hazards when they are unduly apathetic.

- Outrage management ("Calm down!"): How to reassure people about minor hazards when they are unduly upset.
- Crisis communication ("We'll get through it together!"): How to guide people through serious hazards when they are appropriately upset (or even in denial).[7]

By blending the work of Nowak with the plan set forth by the risk communicators, the improved "Ten Step Playbook" is available to get the nation ready for the coming pandemic.

Step 1: Start where your audience is

Officials are advised to start with empathy. Instead of scolding people for their lack of concern, make "common cause with the public" and then talk about how horrible the pandemic is likely to be. Don't tell them the answer; lead them to the conclusion.

Step 2: Don't be afraid to frighten people

Sandman and Lanard advise that "fear appeals have had bad press, but the research evidence that they work is overwhelming." That said, they advise, "We can't scare people enough about H5N1."

Step 3: Acknowledge uncertainty

Sandman gives an example of a senior veterinary official from Thailand's public health department who stated, "We know it is H5, but we're hoping it won't be H5N1," as an example of two additional risk communication principles: acknowledge uncertainty and don't overly reassure. The CDC has been saying since the 1980s that we are "way overdue" for another pandemic. The mass media has apparently been given a green light to magnify this latest health concern by creating ominous warnings with headlines way out of proportion to the risks.

Step 4: Share dilemmas

In crisis communication, the intent of dilemma sharing is to humanize the organization making the decisions and give people the impression they are participating in the planning process. Successful use of this strategy will "reduce the outrage if you turn out to be wrong."

Step 5: Give people things to do

In January 2005, Canadian infectious disease expert Richard Schabas told *The Wall Street Journal,* "Scaring people about avian influenza accomplishes nothing, because we're not asking people to do anything about it." The author's suggestion for giving people something to do includes making a plan for catastrophic, global business disruptions. They even suggest having "cognitive and emotional rehearsals—learning about H5N1 and thinking about what a pandemic might be like and how to cope."

Practicing for disaster is meant to give a "sense of empowerment," but may have little practical value. (The images of school children hiding under their desks during nuclear drills in the 1950s comes to mind.) In addition, nearly every religious tradition and many researchers, including Drs. Deepak Chopra, Larry Dossey, Wayne Dyer, and Pastor Joel Osteen have defined a consistent, clear message: "You get what you think about." Could collective, global "cognitive and emotional rehearsals," anticipating the worst case for the disaster, actually make the situation happen? Perhaps visualizing a safe, clean, healthy world, free of all illnesses for humans, birds, and animals, is a better form of "cognitive rehearsal."

Steps 6, 7, and 8 are specific suggestions on how warnings should stress the magnitude of the coming calamity, focusing on "how bad things could get."

Step 9, "Guide the adjustment reaction," boils down to using the information to manipulate people into a place called a "new normal," one of continual concern and impending doom.

Steps 6 through 9 serve to accentuate Step 2: Don't be afraid to frighten people. Get people revved up. Make them really worried. Get them motivated to fear the coming pandemics: stockpile drugs, push for vaccines, and store water and food. We didn't see a disaster at the millennium—or with swine flu or with smallpox—but a global environmental disaster is just around the next corner. Pass laws to protect the public. Call out the military. It's coming any minute. Soon. We're due. We're doomed.

The last step, Step 10, is to "Inform the public early and aim for total candor and transparency." Sandman argues that it's almost impossible for the government to be too candid and warns against declining to answer questions by using the "security excuse." These last suggestions are the most difficult for governments to adopt, especially in the U.S. The government has collaborated with its agencies to hide so many things from its citizens—from vaccine cover-ups about thimerosal to known problems about Vioxx™—that it has lost trustworthiness.

Do government officials have the ability to be "transparent"?

Crying wolf

On October 20, 2005, the CDC director, Dr. Julie Gerberding, returned from a 10-day avian flu "fact-finding trip" in Asia saying she feared a backlash for "crying wolf" if the flu pandemic doesn't materialize in the near future. Gerberding, who was accompanied by Secretary of Health and Human Services Michael Leavitt and other public health officials, voiced concerns about the "precarious downside" of overly raising the international alarms about the dangers of avian flu. "We're focusing a lot of attention on avian influenza," she said. "But [human-to-human transmission of the disease] hasn't happened—and it may not happen." Gerberding stated that the avian flu may turn out to be a repeat of the 1977 swine flu scare, or it may become the medical equivalent of the "millennium bug" that was widely expected to paralyze the world's computer networks at the beginning of 2000.[8]

Is this government transparency?

More likely she is using the new playbook as a guide, carefully following Step 6: Give warnings that include worst-case scenarios and "always acknowledge that it could turn out to be wrong."[9] Gerberding has reasons to hedge: One of her predecessors at the CDC, Dr. David Sencer, lost his job over the swine flu fiasco. If she doesn't follow the rules—and watch her back—her job could be the next one on the chopping block.

Now that the new plan is out in the open, be mindful of the rhetoric. Pay attention—the news stations and government press releases are playing straight by the book. Even though the "world-saving" bird flu vaccine is clearly more than a year away from release, watch for the upcoming "normal" flu seasons to be the launching pad for a new—and quite possibly mandatory—flu shot that may be coming.

No one should approach the temple of science with
the soul of a money changer.
~Thomas Browne, English Physician and Writer

Chapter 7: Vaccines: A Short Summary of a Long History

Starting points:
- The smallpox vaccine—where it all began
- Current economics of vaccination

To fully understand the vaccine business, a brief review of the history of vaccination is in order. The industry evolved from surprisingly modest origins. When smallpox outbreaks were marching across much of Europe, Englishman Edward Jenner noticed that most milkmaids seemed to escape its ravages. (Jenner, a country apothecary, had purchased his medical degree from St. Andrews University in Scotland for the sum of 15 pounds.) His was an easy observation: Milkmaids boasted blemish-free complexions while smallpox survivors were conspicuous with their facial pockmarks. This led to Jenner's deduction that the milkmaids were somehow protected from the disease, perhaps because they had contracted a milder version of the illness, known as cowpox, from milking the cows.

In 1796, Jenner tested his theory by injecting cowpox pus from Sarah Nelmes, a milkmaid, into James Phipps, a healthy eight-year-old boy. Jenner repeatedly injected Phipps with cowpox pus over several days, gradually increasing the dosage. He then injected Phipps with smallpox and the boy became ill. After a few days, he made a full recovery with no apparent effects from the smallpox or side effects from the vaccine. The experiment was considered a success and the seeds of an industry were sown. Down through history, Jenner has been given credit as the "father of vaccination."[1]

The 19th and 20th centuries saw the introduction of many vaccinations designed to combat infectious diseases. The rewards, in terms of both finances and historical acclaim, were noteworthy. Names like Pasteur, creator of the rabies vaccine, and Salk, developer of the first polio vaccine, are routinely mentioned with the same lofty adoration as Newton and Edison. Since Jenner's introduction 200 years ago, more than 16 childhood and adult vaccines have been put into broad international use. And many more—perhaps as many as 200—are currently under development, illustrating how vaccination has become part of the accepted standards of medicine around the world.

Approximate Development Dates of Vaccines Used in the U.S. (through Feb. 2005)

1798 Smallpox	1935 Yellow Fever	1970 Rubella
1885 Rabies	1945 Influenza	1991 Hepatitis B
1896 Plague (Typhoid)	1955 Injectable Polio	1991 H.flu, (HiB®)
1901 Diptheria	1962 Oral Polio	1995 Chickenpox
1926 Pertussis	1963 Measles	1999 Menomune® (college meningitis)
1927 Tuberculosis, Tetanus	1967 Mumps	2000 Prevnar

During the initial period of production and use, vaccines were largely confined to industrialized countries. Coverage, even in those countries, was patchy because–although the smallpox vaccine was offered to all age groups–only those at risk, mostly healthcare workers and travelers, were aggressively targeted. Despite the accolades given the vaccine for its role in eradicating smallpox, it has been estimated that only about 10 percent of the world's population ever received it. As stated previously, Dr. Tom Mack's opinion was that *"even without mass vaccination,* smallpox would have died out anyway. It was already on its way out. It just would have taken longer." [Emphasis added.][2]

After World War II, while the development of vaccines rapidly increased in scope, the focus was primarily on childhood diseases. With the full endorsement of the U.S. federal government, the implementation of the National Immunization Program was met with nearly universal approval. The future seemed bright for vaccine makers. By 1967, there were 26 companies supplying the U.S. market with various vaccines. By late 2004, the number of major vaccine producers had shrunk to six.

Current economics of vaccination

Of the $347 billion global pharmaceutical market, $8 billion (about 2.5 percent) is represented by sales of all vaccines. Although a tidy sum, consider that in 2004 sales for Lipitor®, Pfizer's cholesterol-lowering medication, weighed in with $10.86 billion. By contrast, the vaccine industry's revenue champ, Prevnar®, given to prevent pneumonia and ear infections in children, had sales of just over $1 billion that same year.

Because vaccines have relatively slim margins and overall profits, the manufacturers have been known to refer to the vaccine sector as the "charity work" of the industry.[3] However, drug companies are driven by money and profits for their shareholders, not charity. A better description for vaccines is they are business "loss leaders," products sold at a substantial discount–or even at a loss–in order to generate sales of another product. With so many children and adults being vaccinated and becoming ill after receiving a vaccine with conditions such as asthma, allergies, ADD/ADHD, eczema, and others—conditions that have been linked to vaccines in medical literature although continually denied by vaccine pundits–perhaps

> The current vaccine manufacturers are Chiron, Merck, GlaxoSmithKline (GSK), Sanofi-Aventis, Wyeth, and MedImmune. Two others, BioPort and Vaxgen, manufacture anthrax vaccine exclusively for the military.

the real profits are in the sale of drugs needed to treat problems caused by vaccines.

The money, it should always be remembered, is in the *medicine*—not the *cure*.

One explanation for this comparatively small market share is that prescription drugs are taken day after day, whereas most vaccinations are given in a short series. Some are given only once or twice in a lifetime. What keeps sales going is the continuous supply of new customers—primarily children. Over the three-year period from 2000 to 2002, the U.S. Bureau of Statistics counted just over four million live births per year. That's an average of 77,500 babies—government-guaranteed customers for vaccines—*each week*. Adding the influenza vaccine to the recommended list of shots for babies, which is now recommended to be given at six months of age and annually thereafter for the rest of a child's life, has certainly expanded the market share for flu shots.

The disdain many people feel for the vaccine companies goes far beyond the short-term pain caused by the jab of a needle. Vaccines have been associated with serious injuries, attested to by the more than 200,000 reports filed with the Vaccine Adverse Event Reporting System (VAERS) since 1994. And, in spite of what authoritative government agencies have declared, thousands of parents have reason to blame vaccines for causing the health problems of their children, ranging from asthma and allergies to diabetes, autism, and even death. Although the CDC, the IOM, and the vaccine manufacturers claim that vaccine reactions are rare—perhaps one or two per million"—if your child is affected, that rare phenomenon is 100 percent to you.

The Pharma-Congress dance: Follow the money

Business schools devote entire courses to consumer psychology. But whatever the clever angle an institution's marketing division may choose, a few simple truths apply to any business. Chief among these is that, while customers pay for products or services in the literal sense, they actually buy something to get a benefit, satisfy a need, or fulfill a demand.

When carpenters buy drill bits, they're really buying *holes.*

Travelers pay for airplane tickets, but they are really buying *transportation.*

Women buy cosmetics, but they are actually satisfying a *need* to project a healthy glow, to cover a blemish, or to *recover lost youth.*

Vaccine manufacturers need to do the same: Provide a benefit, fill a need, or meet a new demand such as the creation of a new product for a particular market niche. However, the misinterpretation of a market demand can send a company into full retreat. The vaccine maker MedImmune experienced the full force of what misjudging a perceived need can do to sales and profits.

According to information presented at the May 2003 National Influenza Summit, approximately 85 percent of Americans between the ages of 20 and 50 go unvaccinated, and nearly 66 percent between the ages of 50 and 64 do not receive the flu vaccine. Assuming that the low influenza vaccination rates are due to an aversion to shots, MedImmune anticipated its pain-free, intranasal vaccine FluMist™ would be a smashing success. MedImmune expected its vaccine to become the next blockbuster drug and anticipated sales to generate revenues of more than $1 billion per year. Every pharma industry watcher agreed it would be a booming success. In fact, on November 7, 2003, FluMist was awarded a prize by *Popular Science* for being one of the best new healthcare products of 2003.[4]

Hundreds of television and print advertisements were designed to persuade consumers to take the "FluMist plunge," squirting a drop of influenza vaccine up their nose instead of getting a needle in the arm. The "most intense, direct-to-consumer marketing campaign ever waged for a vaccine" cost an estimated $25 million over two-and-one-half months.[5] Wyeth, MedImmune's then partner, planned a three-year $100 million campaign to "encourage use of the nasal flu vaccine among physicians." Print advertisements, magazine articles, and rebate coupons from the FluMist website were all part of the blitz. Scare tactics were employed similar to those used while promoting the smallpox vaccine, which warned of the high possibility of a "bioterror attack using the flu virus".[6]

It was all for naught. The first season for FluMist was a

resounding flop. Even when the initial price of $70 per dose was reduced by more than 50 percent, no one wanted the vaccine. Rather than selling its anticipated four to six million doses, MedImmune acknowledged that sales after the launch were as low as 80,000 doses. By the end of November 2003, MedImmune's stock price (as high as $42 a share when it first received FDA approval) plummeted to a 52-week low of $23.40. Obviously, misinterpreting market demand can be both costly and embarrassing.

The vaccine manufacturers claim they have a minimal interest in developing vaccines because there are marginal profits. However, given the potential market share for the global pandemic vaccine, the manufacturers have perked up their collective ears. Every government in the world seems to want the vaccine, and with the current global population at just under 6.5 billion, this vaccine could become a huge economic winner. Each person would require two flu shots: one to "sensitize" the immune system to the new influenza antigen and the second to "induce immunity." Even if prices were as low as $1 per dose, assuming everyone wanted or would be required to get the vaccine, this would increase the sector's gross sales to $13 billion—a 61.5 percent increase over current sales. And that would be in just the first year.

But manufacturers knew from experience that appropriate funding and mandatory insurance safeguards must be set up first in order to proceed. To get these elements in place, Congress needed to be persuaded, and drug companies had the tools to get the job done.

As reported in *Contingencies,* a bi-monthly trade journal for the actuarial profession, the pharmaceutical industry spent $759 million on government lobbying activities between January 1, 1998, and June 20, 2004. The industry reportedly spent more money than any other sector during that period, followed by insurance companies ($644 million) and electric utilities ($588 million). In 2003 alone, lobbying by the pharmaceutical industry amounted to $143 million to promote passage of the Medicare Modernization Act, one of the most significant changes to the 40-year-old Medicare program, and a windfall for years to come for drug sales.[7]

Lobbyists have lavished hundreds of millions of dollars on Congress to ensure that every part of the vaccine development process is in place for the new bird flu vaccine: development grants, tax credits, advanced purchase commitments, and, most importantly, laws that absolve the companies from all product liability issues that may arise from use of an unsafe product.

May we assume, therefore, that chicken cell substrate vaccines are safe?
With biological products, as with crossing the street,
there is no such thing as absolute safety.
~Robin A. Weiss, University College London, U.K.

Chapter 8: Influenza Vaccines: What's in That Needle?

Starting points:
- Making the "regular" flu shot
- Post-egg production: What's in that shot?
- What else is in those eggs?
- Extra viruses in the influenza vaccine and cancer concerns

The method for manufacturing the pandemic vaccine is only slightly different than the steps used to make the influenza vaccine that is produced each year. Some background about the process will provide an understanding of how both the flu shot and the pandemic vaccine currently in development are produced.

The "regular" flu shot

Each year, between January and March, an FDA advisory panel selects the three influenza strains that are expected to be in circulation during the upcoming flu season. Admitting that the process is an "educated guess," the CDC sends the selected seed virus to the FDA for approval prior to distributing the viruses to the manufacturers for production.

The annual flu shot contains three separate strains: two influenza A strains and one strain of influenza B. Most commonly, two of the strains are the same viruses that had been in the preceding year's shot. A third, new strain, is selected each year and then modified in the lab through the reassortment process before it is added to the seasonal shot.

The new strain expected to hit the population during the upcoming season and a second influenza virus known to grow well in eggs are injected into fertilized chicken eggs. The genes from the two viruses "mix together" forming as many as 256 newly created genetic combinations. Researchers select the virus for the vaccine that has both the (H) antigen from the upcoming year's virus and the internal genes from the virus that grows well in eggs. That new, lab-created virus, is added to the two strains from the previous year, to make the vaccine for the current season.[1]

The next few manufacturing steps can be tricky. Vaccine production is a slow, cumbersome process utilizing 500,000 fertilized chicken eggs per day for up to eight months. The two primary manufacturers of the influenza vaccine for the U.S. market, Chiron and Sanofi-Aventis, order hundreds of millions of eggs that become "mini-incubators" for the cultured viruses. The first step of the process involves a labor-intensive method known as "candling"—examining by hand each and every egg with a specialized light. This process allows for the handler to discard any eggs that have not been fertilized, are not growing, or have cracks in the shell.

When the embryo in the fertilized egg is 11 days old, selected eggs are labeled with identification numbers and placed into a tray with the blunt end up. The shells are cleaned using a 70 percent ethanol wipe, and a tiny tuberculin needle is used to punch a small hole into the shell over the air sac. The amniotic membrane of the chicken embryo (the egg white) is then injected with a drop of viral-containing solution. Enough solution is contained in each syringe to inoculate three eggs before the syringe is discarded. The puncture hole in the egg is sealed with a spot of glue, and eggs are maintained for two to three days in a controlled environment between 91.4°F and 93.2°F (33°C and 34°C). During that time, the viruses infect the lungs of the developing chicken embryo and begin to replicate rapidly.

Several days later the eggs are placed into a cooler and chilled to

39°F (3.8°C) overnight. The next day sterile forceps are used to chip open the shell, and the fluid from the three similarly inoculated eggs is collected into a test tube. The gooey viral suspension must be centrifuged—sometimes more than once—to remove as much chicken blood and tissue solution as possible. Some residual egg proteins frequently remain within the final product. Hence, those persons with an egg allergy are strongly advised against receiving the flu shot.

After this "purification" step, a test is performed to detect the presence of an active form of the virus; if none is detected, the specimen is discarded. If virus is present, the solution is submitted for further chemical processing before it is placed into ampoules for sale. The entire process, from egg selection to viral harvest, can take at least six months.[2]

Post-egg production: From the egg to the needle

After the viruses are separated from the egg, they are inactivated (killed) with **formaldehyde,** a known carcinogen. The surface antigens, (H) and (N), are then split by a detergent called **Triton® X-100.** The process spreads the surface antigens apart, increasing the probability of developing an antibody response. Traces of Triton X-100, made by Dow Chemical, can remain in the vaccine solution. Product information on this compound states the following: "Excellent detergent, dispersant, and emulsifier for oil-in-water systems. Uses: Household & industrial cleaners, paints & coatings, pulp & paper, textile, agrochemical, metal working fluids, oil field chemicals."[3]

The suspension of viruses and chemicals is further concentrated in a centrifuge using a **sucrose** (table sugar) solution and then suspended in sodium phosphate-buffered isotonic salt solution. In one of the final steps, a 0.05 percent concentration of **gelatin** is added as a stabilizer, and in many cases, **thimerosal,** the mercury-based preservative, is still added to the multidose vials of the flu vaccine.[4]

Some types of influenza vaccines also include 500 micrograms of **gentamicin,** a broad-spectrum antibiotic, added during the production process to inhibit the growth of bacteria that may be in the suspension. Two other chemicals, **tri-butylphosphate** and **polysorbate 80,** often become part of the "chemical soup" in the vaccine. Tri-butylphosphate is a detergent and polysorbate 80, also known as Tween80™, is an emulsifier. Both are used to disrupt the surface of the virus, making the (H) and (N) antigens more accessible to the immune system. **Resin** is added ostensibly to eliminate substantial portions of these chemicals, but, undoubtedly, residuals of these chemicals remain in the vaccine when injected.

By the time the flu shot is ready for packaging, the solution contains the following: various egg proteins, Triton-X100, formaldehyde, resin, gelatin, tri-butylphosphate, polysorbate 80, and, in some instances, gentamicin. To preserve this chemical brew in doses of up to 25 micrograms, thimerosal (a mercury derivative) is still added to many of the shots.

After reading this vivid description of the manufacture of the influenza vaccine, the thought of injecting this into your body—or the body of your baby—should be repugnant.

For those not repulsed by the idea of injecting the above solution into your body, perhaps knowing that the vaccine won't prevent you from getting the flu will add to your perspective. A report released by the *Cochrane Collaboration* in January 2006 concluded that there was no evidence that injecting children six to 23 months of age with the influenza vaccine was any more effective than a placebo in preventing the flu. After a review of 51 studies involving more than 260,000 children, including 17 papers translated from Russian, the co-author of the study and coordinator of the Rome-based Cochrane Vaccine Project, Dr. Thomas Jefferson, concluded that mandates to vaccinate babies is based on very little evidence that the shot will keep them healthy during the flu season.[5]

Furthermore, the reviewers found no evidence to back claims that vaccines prevent deaths from influenza or other serious complications in this age group. As for "safety studies," there aren't any. "We were astonished to find only one safety study of inactivated vaccine in children under two years of age; that was carried out nearly 30 years ago and only in 35 children," stated Dr. Jefferson.[6]

Jefferson went on to strongly chide the governments of Canada and the U.S. for their mass vaccination policies, stating, "Research should be done before anybody makes a decision, not afterward. Otherwise, you're in the business of experimenting with your population."[7]

Also released in January 2006 by the *Cochrane Collaboration* was a report that determined the results for vaccinating healthy adults were equally as dismal. Twenty-five reports of studies involving nearly 60,000 people were included. Overall, vaccination reduced the risk of influenza by only 6 percent and negligibly reduced the average number of missed work days (by 0.16 days). The reviewers concluded that universal immunization of healthy adults was not supported by the results of the review.[8]

The *Cochrane Collaboration* is the same organization that concluded that the effectiveness of flu shots, particularly in the elderly, was "wildly overstated," as reported in *The New York Times* on September 21, 2005. So, the flu shot is not effective in babies, its effectiveness in the elderly is "wildly overstated," and it is not recommended for healthy adults. By any measure, that is just about everyone.

Keep these studies in mind as the hype for mass vaccination begins. Understand that the new bird flu vaccine will be experimental, it will have no proof of safety, will lack efficacy and should be avoided.

And what else is in those eggs?

Eggs used in the production of the influenza vaccine are purchased by the tens of millions each season. But what's in those eggs?

An entire industry has evolved for the purpose of providing eggs for vaccine research and production. Produced by specific pathogen-free (SPF) flocks, the birds have been certified to be free of contamination from *certain* microorganisms. The chickens are raised vaccine-free in isolated, air-filtered buildings that are expensive to maintain, making the cost of SPF eggs more expensive than eggs available at the supermarket. The designation of SPF is used to refer to these birds, which are tested frequently to ensure that the "microbiological integrity" of the flock is maintained; meaning the viruses and the bacteria in the birds remain the same.

In addition to testing the birds, their eggs are also closely inspected to maintain and guarantee their specific pathogen-free status. The eggs are tested for a list of viruses and bacteria—usually between 25 and 37—to confirm the absence of specific pathogens on the list. If none of the listed agents are detected, the egg is reported as "pathogen free."[9]

However, that is not necessarily the case.

The number of viruses and/or bacteria that eggs are screened for is finite, even though there are an abundance of potential agents from which to choose. To screen for every microbe would be completely time- and cost-prohibitive. So in theory, *if* human vaccines are made from SPF eggs, and *if* the standards of Good Manufacturing Practice are maintained, vaccines *should* be specific pathogen-free and safe for human use with little concern of cross-species contamination.

The truth is, each egg is a new experiment.

Disturbingly, there is a wide difference between *"specific pathogen-free"* eggs and *"pathogen free"* eggs. The distinction is so important that in its July 1996 report, the Institutes of Medicine (IOM) acknowledged that "although it is not possible to produce a completely uncontaminated animal, it is possible to produce an animal [or egg] certified to be *free of specific pathogens.*"[10]

Could unidentified pathogens be present in eggs and be passed into the finished product of the current—and the future pandemic—influenza vaccines? Could viruses that are harmless to their animal host be dangerous to humans? This grave concern is more than theoretical because harmful extra viruses have been passed on in vaccines before.

Over the last 15 to 20 years, researchers have recorded a litany of serious disease-causing transmissions through vaccines. In the 1940s, hepatitis B was transmitted via the albumen used to stabilize the yellow fever vaccine.[11] Between 1955 and 1962, at least a third of all polio vaccines were thought to be contaminated with the cancer-causing virus SV40.[12] Similarly, human blood products, blood-derived materials, and clotting factors have transmitted infectious agents through extra viruses. Both hepatitis C and paravirus B-19 have been passed to hemophiliacs through contaminated products.[13]

Because eggs are currently used for the manufacture of several vaccines other than influenza—measles, mumps, and yellow fever—and will most likely be used for the production of the new H5N1 vaccine, the potential for continued contamination is real. The chart provided by Charles River Laboratories is an example of infectious agents that eggs are commonly tested for. If these viruses are absent from the eggs, they are labeled SPF eggs. Given the hundreds of known viruses and bacteria with which they could be contaminated, this list is dangerously short.[14]

Egg Grade Comparison

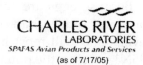

CHARLES RIVER
LABORATORIES
SPAFAS Avian Products and Services
(as of 7/17/05)

Agent	Antigen	Test	Premium	Premium Plus	Research
Avian Adenovirus Group I - Celo Type I	CELO-Phelps	AGP	X	X	X
Avian Adenovirus Group II (HEV)	Domermuth	AGP	X	X	X
Avian Adenovirus Group III (EDS)	CLKK115D	HI	X	X	X
Avian Encephalomyelitis	van Roekel	ELISA, AGP	X	X	X
Avian Influenza (Type A)	T/W/66	ELISA, AGP	X	X	X
Avian Nephritis Virus	G4260	IFA	X	X	X
Avian Paramyxovirus Type 2	Yucaipa	HI	X	X	X
Avian Reovirus	S 1133	ELISA, AGP, IFA	X	X	X
Avian Rhinotracheitis Virus	UK	ELISA	X	X	X
Avian Rotavirus	Ch-2	AGP	X	X	X
Avian Tuberculosis	M. avium	CO, PM	X	X	X
Chicken Anemia Virus	DelRose	IFA		X	X
Endogenous GS Antigen	p27	ELISA			X
Fowl Pox	Conn	AGP, CO	X	X	X
Hemophilus paragallinarum	Serovars A,B,C	CO	X	X	X
Infectious Bronchitis - Ark.	Ark 99	ELISA, HI	X	X	X
Infectious Bronchitis - Conn.	Conn A5968	ELISA, HI	X	X	X
Infectious Bronchitis - JMK	JMK	ELISA, HI	X	X	X
Infectious Bronchitis - Mass.	Mass 66579	ELISA, HI	X	X	X
Infectious Bursal Disease	M4040(2512)	ELISA, AGP, SN	X	X	X
Infectious Laryngotracheitis	UC A92430	ELISA, AGP, SN	X	X	X
Lymphoid Leukosis A, B	RSV-RAV A,B	MNT	X	X	X
Lymphoid Leukosis Viruses	A,B,C,D,E,J	ELISA	X	X	X
Marek's Disease (Serotypes 1,2, 3)	SB-1	AGP	X	X	X
Mycoplasma gallisepticum	A5969	SPA	X	X	X
Mycoplasma synoviae	WVU 1853	SPA	X	X	X
Newcastle Disease	LaSota	ELISA, AGP, HI	X	X	X
Reticuloendotheliosis Virus	ATCC 770 T	IFA, AGP	X	X	X
Salmonella pullorum-gallinarum	K Polyvalent	SPA	X	X	X
Salmonella species		IA	X	X	X

AGP=Agar Gel Preipitin
CO=Clinical Observation
ELISA=Enzyme-Linked Immunosobent Assay
HI=Hemagglutination Inhibition
IA=Isolation of Agent

MNT=Microneutralization
SN=Serum Neutralization
SPA=Serum Plate Agglutination
TA=Tube Agglutination
PM=Post Mortem

Chart provided by Charles River Laboratories. Reproduced with permission.

Extra viruses in the influenza vaccines

One virus that has garnered a great deal of attention because of its confirmed presence in vaccines is called endogenous avian leucosis virus, or ALV. Nearly 45 years ago it was found that apparently healthy hens could transmit ALV to their eggs and then to vaccines. Found in all chicken cell lines, ALV is known to infect large segments of the modern poultry industry and because it is found in all commercial chickens and eggs, humans are exposed on a consistent basis.

ALV is considered a "parent" virus because it can easily transform into other potentially cancer-causing sarcoma viruses. A short list is included here for scientific minds:

- Avian myeloblastosis virus;
- Avian myelocytoma virus;
- Avian erythroblastosis virus;
- Fujinami sarcoma virus;
- many other sarcoma viruses.

Sarcoma viruses are retroviruses; these types of viruses have been shown to cause cancer. One group of researchers who studied the actions of ALV wrote, "Serial passage of a retrovirus that does not carry an oncogene leads with high frequency to the emergence of new viruses that have transduced oncogenes...." That is professional double-speak for the following: Given the right conditions, ALV can easily transform into other viruses known to be cancer-related.[15]

Another virus discovered in 1985 is called endogenous avian retrovirus or EAV—a known contaminant of influenza vaccines. This virus is present in all breeds of chicken and cannot be eliminated from even the most stringently kept flocks.[16] EAV has an associated enzyme called *reverse transcriptase.* The job of this enzyme is to copy the genetic material of the virus from RNA into DNA, reversing the flow of genetic information, which is normally copied from DNA into RNA. Since 1982, researchers have identified the presence of EAV and reverse transcriptase in influenza vaccines.[17]

As recently as 1999, a research team led by Shirley Tsang, detected the presence of reverse transcriptase in the measles and mumps vaccines.[18] They tracked the enzyme's origin back to the chicken cells the viruses had been grown in. Considering the numerous regulations requiring all avian cell cultures to be free of known chicken viruses, this was an alarming discovery and should have set off alarms throughout the scientific and medical communities. Because of the way reverse transcriptase works in living cells, it is possible that genetic material from chicken viruses is being woven into human DNA, particularly the DNA of children.[19]

That is a sobering thought.

But like so many other concerns about vaccine safety that should cause the industry to snap to attention, researchers are focused on proving that the adventitious (extra) viruses are benign rather than admitting they exist and searching for evidence that they may be causing harm.

Avian virus contamination and cancer

The issue of chicken virus contamination is discussed regularly by government agencies that regulate the production of egg-based vaccines. The CDC, the FDA, the Center for Biologics Evaluation and Research (CBER), and other branches of the public health service have convened on many occasions to discuss the implications of the potential vaccine contaminants.

In a workshop co-sponsored by the FDA and the CBER, named "Evolving Scientific and Regulatory Perspectives on Cell Substrates for Vaccine Development," held on September 10, 1999, experts gathered from government and industry to once again discuss the problems of vaccine contaminants. Dr. Phil Minor from the National Institute of Biological Standards and Control (NIBSC)—the CBER equivalent in the United Kingdom—was the first speaker of the morning of the meeting's sixth session. Minor gave a straightforward introduction, voicing concerns over the problem of animal viruses contaminating human vaccines.

After the customary opening remarks, Minor related that the most serious contaminations in vaccines came from materials derived from whole animal sources. He went on to explain that eggs used in the production of influenza vaccines are counted as "animal," as defined by the Animal Regulated Use Act in the U.K., "because they are embryonated" (i.e., they have been fertilized and the embryo has started to grow).[20]

There is little argument among researchers that avian retroviruses and reverse transcriptase have long been detected in influenza vaccines and other vaccines made from eggs. What they do *not* agree upon, however, are the effects these extra viruses may be having on humans, including the possibility that they may be causing cancer.

The extra viruses in the vaccines are considered to be completely benign by some researchers. These contaminants, called "free riders," have not been found to interact in any way with the immune system or other cells of the vaccine recipient. However, considering all contaminants to be completely benign has a glaring flaw: Even though many *inactive* viruses have been tested and are indeed harmless, not *all* viruses have been tested. If some are found to be *active*—meaning, they have the ability to replicate—they could very well cause harm.

Attempting to determine the effects of viral contaminants on humans has an added complexity. Part of the normal lifecycle of a retrovirus involves integrating, for a variable period, into the host's DNA. The virus can insert itself and become invisible to the immune system–beyond the reach of antibodies to detect and remove it. This also means the virus is beyond the scope of the researcher's testing tools to find it.[21]

If a virus isn't detected, it is considered by scientists to be absent. Lack of detection, however, is not proof that the viruses are not causing harm. Researchers may have difficulty identifying the presence of retroviruses in human serum through advanced testing because the virus' genetic material may already be incorporated into human DNA.

Chicken cell cultures are not the only concern for adventitious (extra) viral contaminants found in vaccines. Another animal source, bovine sera from calves, is used for the production of the following vaccines: rubella, chickenpox, polio, Prevnar, and the adult pneumonia shot. Nearly 100 percent of this commercially available serum obtained from cows is contaminated with bovine viruses. The point of this discussion is to ask the following question: Are we incorporating viruses from chickens and cows into the human genome? Are we altering the genes of future generations in unknown ways through vaccines?

A well-researched, highly documented paper published online by an obvious industry insider, going by the name of Benjamin McReardon, describes in detail the problem of not knowing whether a viral gene is active or inactive. If active, ALV viruses may have the capacity to activate cancer-causing genes in the host's cells:

> "Considering that ALV can, for example, easily capture the human oncogenes [called] "erbB" and "myc," and these two oncogenes are strongly associated with common forms of **human breast cancer,** it seems that the issue of ALV vaccine contamination should deserve a high level of attention....A well-known microbiology text reinforces these concepts by teaching, "Proto-oncogenes become incorporated into retroviral genomes with surprising ease." [Emphasis added.][22]

It has been said that the seeds of cancer lie within us. The human genome contains at least 50 genes called proto-oncogenes, which under normal conditions maintain a watchful eye over excessive cell division and keep it under control. However, when these genes become "activated" (i.e., when a proto-oncogene is converted into an active oncogene), uncontrolled cell growth can occur. Activation of a proto-oncogene can be caused by a variety of mechanisms including the insertion of viral DNA or RNA into the host's genome. When cells undergo rapid, unchecked cell division, the possibility for abnormal cells to arise and replicate is more than a theoretical concern. This is the start of cancer.

The effects on the global population

The medical literature documents the presence of viral

contaminants found within the influenza vaccine. If the flu shot were given only once in a lifetime, perhaps the load of additional chicken viruses delivered in a single shot would have minimal consequences. But the influenza vaccine is now recommended for infants starting at six months of age and is intended to be given annually for the rest of that child's life. Could potentially cancer-causing retroviruses and other viruses be incorporated into a child's genome without detection, leading to health problems later in life? It's not an unreasonable question.

As reported on May 9, 2002, by Samuel S. Epstein, MD, chairman of the Cancer Prevention Coalition and professor emeritus of Environmental and Occupational Medicine, University of Illinois School of Public Health, Chicago, the incidence of childhood cancer has steadily increased. He notes that, ironically, since passage of the 1971 National Cancer Act, which launched the "War Against Cancer," childhood cancer has risen by 26 percent. The incidence of particular forms of childhood cancer has increased even more than the average: acute lymphocytic leukemia (ALL), 62 percent; brain cancer, 50 percent; and bone cancer, 40 percent.[23]

Certainly, a laundry list of environmental causes has been implicated in the exponential rise in cancer in children: Paternal and maternal exposures to occupational carcinogens, such as dioxin; exposures to pesticides in the home, including pet flea collars, and lawn and garden products; consumption of nitrites in meat; and even treatment with Ritalin for attention deficit disorders may pose risks of causing rare, highly aggressive liver cancers.[24]

But one has to wonder: Does early exposure to vaccines that contain adventitious, contaminating viruses, reverse transcriptase, and other toxic vaccine ingredients injected multiple times into infants less than one year of age lay the groundwork for cancer as children grow into adulthood?

What's at stake

The risk of incorporating retroviruses into human DNA have

gone up substantially since 2004 when the influenza vaccine was added to the pediatric schedule, targeting six to 23-month-old babies. With the specter of pandemic influenza mass vaccination looming on the horizon, more red flags need to be raised. With each egg-based vaccine, the risk that even more avian viruses will be introduced into the human genome goes up exponentially.

The logarithmic increase of exposure to viral contaminants has caught the attention of a few concerned researchers. Dr. Martin Myers from the National Vaccine Program posed a thoughtful question at the previously mentioned September 1999 CBER workshop.[25] Questioning long-term safety, Myers asked, "As I sit and count the number of immunizations that various populations receive with these [retroviral] particles in them, I wonder if there is any data on sero-responsiveness in longitudinal [studies]" (meaning, have we followed these children over an extended period to see if they have developed antibodies to viral contaminants?). An even more appropriate question would have been, "Have we looked for health problems in these children to see if they have been caused by the viral contaminants in these vaccines?"

A response came from James S. Robertson, PhD, from NIBSC. He interrupted Myers, stating, "There is no evidence for any increase in the incidence of childhood cancers since the onset of [the] measles and mumps vaccination program."[26]

This assessment is as incomplete as it is inaccurate.

A more accurate statement would be, "We have not identified any increase in childhood cancer caused by retroviruses," which begs the question: Are researchers actually looking for an association between retroviruses and cancer? You can't find what you're not looking for. Finding an association between retroviruses in vaccines and cancer would be disastrous for the vaccine program. Because no one wants to find this association, funding for this type of research would be hard to come by.

At the end of his own presentation, Dr. Phil Minor again addressed the group, summarizing his concerns this way: ". . . the issues that I have been dealing with really have to do with primary cells and primary cell problems where the virus comes directly from animals. ...there is no doubt in my mind that that is the main source of concern in terms of human health."[27] Keep in mind that by definition an "egg" is an "animal."

His conclusions were echoed by a CDC virologist, Dr. Walid Heneine, also in attendance at the CBER workshop. Dr. Heneine publicly cautioned the importance of not generalizing about the hypothesis that no harm is being caused by the accidental avian viruses in vaccines. She mentioned research conducted in 1997 by Weissmahr, et al., demonstrating that because viral contaminants were capable of replicating, they may be capable of causing harm.[28] In addition, Heneine suggested that "prudence be followed" because even though the presence of some viruses are *known,* other disease-causing viruses may be present although they have not yet been detected.

What's coming through that needle could be deadly.

Today, the NIH is working with vaccine makers to develop new cell-culture techniques that will help us bring a pandemic flu vaccine to the American people faster in the event of an outbreak...and it would allow us to produce enough vaccine for every American in time.
~President G.W. Bush, November 1, 2005

Chapter 9: Beyond Eggs: Cell-Culture Vaccines and Toxic Adjuvants

Starting points:
- New vaccines: From cell lines instead of eggs
- First tested: VERO cells from African green monkey kidneys
- Other cell lines: PER.C6 from human retinas, FluBLOK™ from caterpillar eggs, MDCK from dogs
- New chemicals: MF59

S anofi-Pasteur, the vaccine arm of the mega Sanofi-Aventis Group, has become a mega-partner with the U.S. Department of Health and Human Services. Over the last two years, the company has completed negotiations on five pandemic-related agreements with the U.S. government to produce doses of a trial pandemic vaccine using the H5N1 virus.

The first contract signed in May 2004 was an agreement between Sanofi-Pasteur and NIAID to produce 8,000 investigational doses of H5N1 vaccine for a phase I human clinical trial. The vaccine was manufactured at the Swiftwater, Pennsylvania, facility and used in human trials that took place at three university-based centers throughout the U.S: the University of Rochester, the University of Maryland at Baltimore, and the University of California, Los Angeles. The study, which included 452 healthy adults, was designed to assess the immune response and safety profile of the new experimental vaccine. The results of the three-month trial started to come in at the end of August 2004 and were mixed at best.

As reported in *The New York Times,* a positive antibody response occurred only in 115 of the participants (25.4 percent) with two doses of vaccine given—an initial dose and a second dose given four weeks later. NIAID Director Anthony Fauci was quoted in the *Times* story as saying, "It's good news. We have a vaccine." However, it wasn't *all* good news. In fact, part of the information was dreadful news for the manufacturers. The vaccine required 90 micrograms of viral antigen to elicit an antibody response, and the vaccine had to be given twice—a total of 180 micrograms. This immediately caused a monumental challenge in regard to production capacity. In comparison, the annual flu shot requires only 15 micrograms of viral antigen per shot. "I predict they won't get much immune response at all," said Tony Colegate, head of the industry's pandemic task force for Chiron, U.K.[1]

In a subsequent *Wall Street Journal* report on October 14, 2005, Fauci reported that, based on current results, the two million doses ordered by the U.S. government would only cover about 450,000 people. Infectious disease expert Michael Osterholm, MD, expressed concern over this supply issue, stating that *12 times the amount* of antigen will be needed to get the same response a typical flu shot would trigger.[2]

The conventional explanation for this lackluster response to the H5 antigen is that this new virus has never been "seen" before by the immune system, and the system needs to be "primed" to generate an adequate response. However, this reveals a serious contradiction. If the H5N1 virus is as dangerous to humanity as it is being portrayed in the media, then a small amount of the antigen should generate a huge immunological response. This does not appear to be the case.

A more feasible explanation is that the virus really doesn't present a significant threat to the body after all. This assumption is supported by the *New England Journal of Medicine* article published in September

2005 reporting that even with constant exposure, humans appear to be highly resistant to the problems caused by the virus.[3] It can also account for the thousands of persons who have been exposed to H5N1 but demonstrate only mild disease or no disease at all.

The news that much more antigen would be required to meet vaccine demand meant standard production methods, using the egg-based techniques, would be inadequate. Each factory that manufactures flu shots has a limited production capacity, partially due to space constraints needed to house tens of millions of eggs. In addition, the process requires up to six months to produce a single lot of vaccine. The current methodology has no room for error and no capacity to ramp up production beyond the eggs slotted to be used in a single season. A new type of vaccine production was needed, including new factories. Anticipating this need, Sanofi-Pasteur, manufacturer of the experimental vaccine, was the first to push for the use of a new technology—cell-based influenza vaccines.

First described in the mid-1990s and still in the experimental stages, the new technology has drawn all major players in the vaccine industry into attempts to develop cell culture technology for flu shots. The methodology can be rapidly expanded in times when the government thinks there is an emergency need for any vaccine that is made from eggs.

Although new for flu shots, cell-culture technology is hardly new. It has been used since the 1950s for the production of polio, measles, mumps, and tetanus vaccines. Far different from the tedious egg-based methodology, cell-culture methods grow the viruses in large steel vats filled with living cells. The viruses enter the cells and rapidly replicate, allowing for large-scale harvest of influenza viruses in a matter of days. While the egg-based method requires three to six months to develop the viruses for a vaccine, the cell-based method, from start to finished product, takes approximately 60 days, with five to six viral harvests extracted every three weeks.

Cell-line technology has not been used for flu shots primarily for logistical reasons: It would require a complete retooling of existing production facilities. None of the manufacturers have been willing to invest the hundreds of millions of dollars and the five to seven years required to build new vaccine plants. But with the threat of a pandemic looming on the horizon, the need for hundreds of millions of doses of vaccine, and tens of billions in federal dollars available to fund the capital improvements, the reason and the means are in place to proceed.

Sanofi-Pasteur was the first to access the government's money trough, signing an agreement to build its new cell-based manufacturing facility. On April 1, 2005, Department of Health and Human Services awarded Sanofi-Pasteur a $97 million contract to speed development of its new plant. The five-year grant would help the company quickly revamp its existing manufacturing facility at the Swiftwater location. This site has been producing influenza vaccines for more than 50 years and currently manufactures several versions of the flu shot, including Fluzone®, the only influenza vaccine approved for use in the U.S. for children six to 35 months of age.[4]

The newly renovated, 145,000 square foot (13,470 square meters), $150 million facility is expected to be running at full capacity in time for the 2009 influenza season, and with the help of the government grant it will be completed ahead of schedule. Anticipated to create more than 100 new production jobs, the plant will ultimately be capable of producing at least 300 million doses of influenza vaccine annually—one for every citizen in America.

Egg replacement candidates

Although the idea of growing viruses in eggs to create a vaccine sounds abhorrent to some, the choices for cell line vaccines are no less offensive. As early as 1996, manufacturers began discussing the development of cell line influenza vaccines in anticipation of the impending demand driven by a pandemic. Preliminary studies indicated that VERO cells were a good choice for growing influenza A and B viruses.[5] First used by Salk in the 1950s to produce polio vaccines, VERO cells are derived from the kidneys of African green monkeys. The cells have been under fire for many years due to their potential for serious contamination by an adventitious virus referred to as Simian virus 40 (SV40).

Researcher and assistant professor of pathology at Loyola University in Chicago, Dr. Michele Carbone, has gone head-to-head with the FDA and the NIH for years over his discovery linking SV40 to specific types of human tumors. His research showed that when SV40 was injected into hamsters the same types of tumors developed that had occurred in human cells infected with SV40.[6] Even though these findings may seem to be of only scientific interest, they hold significant implications for public health. SV40 was found to be a contaminant in polio vaccines from 1955 until 1963, resulting in the injection of millions of people with potentially tumor-causing viruses.[7] Using VERO cells for the production of a pandemic influenza vaccine intended for use by every person in the world could have disastrous implications.

As recently as 2002, the CBER was disturbed enough over the carcinogenic potential of VERO cells that it issued a memorandum to manufacturers urging the need for "tumorigenicity testing" (determining the ability of the VERO cells to induce tumors) of each manufacturer's VERO master cell bank. The memo went on to state that, based on extensive internal discussions, consultation with outside experts, and comments received from the Vaccines and Related Biological Products Advisory Committee (VRBPAC) during a meeting held on May 12, 2000, the committee had "residual concerns" it wanted the manufacturers to address—namely, ensuring that the final vaccine products were completely "free of residual intact VERO cells." The CBER memo also acknowledged that, even though the WHO's "acceptable limit" for the number of residual VERO cells per vaccine was ten nanograms per dose, the CBER wanted *all* the cells out. The CBER also wanted the right to assess the cancer-causing risks of each vaccine lot on a "case-by-case basis for all viral vaccines."[8]

That is an overwhelming amount of concern. If the CBER is willing to admit this degree of apprehension over VERO cells, the cancer-causing potential of these cells is obviously immense.

Two years after the precautionary memo was issued, the complications of using VERO cell substrates for the development of an influenza vaccine emerged. In 2002, Baxter Healthcare Corporation had received regulatory approval in the Netherlands to develop a new influenza vaccine, PrefluCel™, using the company's VERO cell technology. Baxter was pursuing regulatory approval for

PrefluCel in other European countries and had plans to initiate clinical trials in the U.S.

However, on December 9, 2004, Baxter announced that it had voluntarily suspended enrollment of participants in its Phase II/III clinical study for PrefluCel due to a higher than expected rate of mild fever and associated symptoms discovered among clinical trial participants. Norbert G. Riedel, Baxter's chief scientific officer, explained, "Based on the preliminary data we've seen, the rate of fever and associated symptoms observed with the current formulation of PrefluCel is higher compared to other vaccines available on the market."[9] The clinical trials were stopped without further explanation, and, to date, no further testing has resumed.

With VERO cells out of the immediate running, the next most likely cell line candidate for the production of the new pandemic flu vaccine is called PER.C6®—cells that have originated from the retina of aborted fetal tissue. The process used to create the PER.C6 cells is complex. It requires extracting normal human retina cells and transforming them into perpetually dividing cells by exposing them to a virus—Adenovirus 5. The resultant cells are labeled "designer substrates." That these cells can be harmful to humans is more than a theoretical consideration. Perpetually dividing cells, by definition, are neoplastic (cancerous) cells. When test animals were injected with the Adenovirus 5 alone, no tumors formed. However, when mice were injected with the Adenovirus-retina cell combined with the designer substrate, tumors began to appear. The FDA is fully aware of this potential problem, as reported in an FDA memo in 2001, but the research and clinical trials have been allowed to continue.[10]

A few other cell lines under consideration

An independent company, Protein Sciences Corporation, has been working to develop a patented influenza vaccine that will be produced from *insect cells.* This vaccine strategy, known commercially as FluBlok®, isolates a purified concentration of the hemagglutinin (H) antigen from the vaccine-bound virus and inserts the (H) antigen into a second virus called a baculovirus. The (H)-containing baculovirus is inserted into caterpillar cells growing in culture. Several Phase I and II trials conducted by NIAID that included more than 600 subjects using FluBlok® demonstrated that the bug-created vaccine elicited a strong antibody response in humans.[11]

One additional cell line under consideration is called Madin-Darby canine kidney cells (MDCK), extracted from the kidneys of a healthy female cocker spaniel in 1958. The cell line has been transformed in the perpetually dividing cells, called "immortalized cells," similar to the PER.C6 cells. Solvay Pharmaceuticals, a Dutch company, has been working with this cell-culture to produce influenza vaccines since the early 1990s, where the cells have been approved for use in the Netherlands. The company, hoping to soon become a serious contender for vaccine production in the U.S., is seeking FDA approval for its dog kidney cell-produced flu vaccine.

Solvay's closest competitor, Chiron, filed an investigational new drug application in 2004 to create influenza vaccines using the MDCK cell line. The experimental vaccine is currently under development in Chiron's flu cell culture manufacturing facility in Marburg, Germany.

The FDA is fully aware that the new cell substrates made from animal tissues come with risks that in many ways are no different from the risks associated with using eggs. The cells can become contaminated with adventitious viruses that are potentially deadly. A recent FDA memo acknowledges the risks:

> "The experience in the early 1960s with SV40 contamination of poliovirus and adenovirus vaccines and the continuing questions regarding whether SV40 could be responsible for some human neoplasms [cancers] underscores the importance of keeping viral vaccines free of adventitious agents [viral contaminants]. This is particularly important when there is a theoretical potential for contamination of a vaccine with viruses that might be associated with neoplasia [cancer].

"It is unclear whether neoplastic cells [cell substrates] have a greater or lower risk [of contamination] than other types of cells....However, if their growth in tissue culture is not well controlled, there may exist additional opportunities for contamination of cells with a longer lifespan."[12]

And it gets worse. The same FDA memo goes on to say:

"In addition to the possibility of contamination of cell substrates...the use of immortalized, neoplastic human cells to develop [vaccines] raises theoretical concerns with regard to possible contamination with TSE/BSE agents."[13]

TSE is Transmissible Spongiform Encephalopathy, a condition that includes a group of rare degenerative brain disorders characterized by tiny holes in the brain tissues, giving a "spongy" appearance when viewed under a microscope. When this condition occurs in cows, it is called Bovine Spongiform Encephalopathy, commonly known as "mad cow disease." In a study published in 2004, researchers found that *any cell line* could potentially support the propagation of TSE agents.[14]

Clearly, CBER, a division of the FDA, is disquieted over the carcinogenic potential of substrate cells and wants manufacturers to take every available step to eliminate them from the vaccine final product. The FDA admits serious concerns about contamination of all types of cell lines. The question that begs an answer is, knowing the cancer-causing potential of the cell lines and the cancer-causing risks of contaminants in the cell lines, why is this technology being promoted? Or better, why is the FDA allowing its use at all? Despite substantial evidence—and even admissions of concern—the FDA appears to be flagrantly ignoring the potential for harm to vaccine recipients through this technology and is recklessly approving the use of these products for the manufacture of the pandemic vaccine.

Stretching the available vaccine

Manufacturers are scrambling to create a pandemic flu vaccine for "every man, woman, and child" in the U.S, a concept first introduced by former head of HHS, Tommy Thompson, when the same manufacturers were scurrying to make the smallpox vaccine.[15]

But even with billions of tax dollars allocated through federal appropriations to grease the wheels, it will be several years before the cell-based flu vaccines are ready for market. In the meantime, makers have contrived a way to stretch the available bird flu vaccine to provide injections for millions more recipients in the event the government announces they are needed—through the addition of vaccine adjuvants.

An adjuvant is a substance added to produce a high antibody response using the smallest amount of viral-containing (antigen) solution possible in the shot. By definition, adjuvants are considered to be "pharmacologically active drugs." They are designed to be "inert without inherent activity or toxicity on their own, yet they are required to potently augment effects of the other compounds" in the vaccines.[16] It is difficult to explain how a substance can be defined as "pharmacologically active" and at the same time be described as "inert and have no activity or toxicity."

The first adjuvants were used in 1925 by French researcher G. Ramon. He found that by adding breadcrumbs, agar, tapioca, starch, or oil lecithin to vaccines, he could increase the antibody response to diphtheria and tetanus antitoxins. Although these substances are no longer used, adjuvants are regularly added to vaccines. They are grouped chemically into "classes" based on their mechanisms of action. For example, hypertensive drugs are grouped together based on the effect they have on the body; one can be classified as a beta-blocker and another as an ace-inhibitor. Adjuvants are similarly grouped based on the type of immune system response they are *thought* to induce. But therein lies the rub: After more than 75 years of use, the mechanism of actions for most adjuvants is still "incompletely understood." In other words, what they do to the body is unknown.[17]

In clinical trials for a new vaccine, animals are injected with live, replicating viruses or bacteria to observe the immune response. Sometimes, the selected organism is so strong it kills the animal. In those instances, the pathogen must first undergo a process called "attenuation" or "weakening" before it can be used in humans. The problem is that even though the dead organisms are considered to be safer, they are often ignored by the immune system. An adjuvant is added to the vaccine for two reasons: (1) to anchor the solution to the injection site for an extended period, allowing the body to recognize that it has been invaded by a foreign substance and send white blood cells to the area to generate a response, and (2) to cause an increased inflammatory response at the site of the injection, resulting in higher levels of antibodies being produced to eliminate and then "remember" the injected pathogen.

For the adjuvant to work, it must be attached to a molecule called a "carrier" or a "vehicle". The combination (adjuvant + carrier) is referred to as an "adjuvant formula", a supposedly inert compound. The combination of the attenuated (dead) virus or bacteria plus the adjuvant formula used in a vaccine causes an amazingly complex immunological cascade of events, including the release of dozens of molecules called cytokines that cause inflammation and activation of the immune response.[18]

The nonspecific response induced by the vaccine and its adjuvant wreaks havoc in the normally organized, highly structured immune system. What happens is rather like setting off a tiny explosion under a pile of dry, fall leaves, watching the explosion, and then trying to describe the trajectory of the leaves by explaining where they landed. Hardly inert, the reaction that occurs within each individual after receiving a vaccine, is truly a new experiment.

Adjuvants have the potential for causing serious health problems. A partial list of risks that have been associated with adjuvants includes the following:[19]

- Local or acute inflammation, including the formation of painful abscesses, persistent nodules, ulcers, or draining lymph nodes;
- Induction of fever, muscle pain, joint pain, and headaches—much like the flu;

- Immune suppression;
- Anaphylaxis (shock), hives, and vasculitis;
- Systemic toxicity to tissues and organs;
- Induction of autoimmune arthritis and other autoimmune disorders;
- Cross-reactivity with human cells, causing glomerulonephritis (renal failure) and meningoencephalitis (brain swelling);
- Genetic events: carcinogenesis (cancer), teratogenesis (birth defects), and abortogenesis (causing abortions)

Choosing an adjuvant for use in humans is difficult because it must be based on the level of toxicity observed when the adjuvant formulation is injected into animals. Decades of experimentation have shown that "successful predictions about safety, potency, or efficacy in humans for a particular adjuvant cannot be reliably made from [animal] models. Unfortunately, the absolute safety of vaccines containing adjuvants, *or any vaccine*, cannot be guaranteed." [Emphasis added.][20]

For decades, vaccine developers have been tinkering with various substances to "trick" the body into producing heightened immune responses, measured as an antibody. The only adjuvants currently licensed for use in humans in North America are aluminum compounds—aluminum sulfate, aluminum hydroxide, and aluminum phosphate—which have been in use since the 1920s. The limiting factor for approval of new adjuvants has been that most are far too toxic for use in humans. However, one adjuvant has been approved in Europe, and approval is on its way for use in the U.S. It is an oil-based adjuvant called MF59, primarily composed of squalene.

On first blush, squalene seems like a good choice for an adjuvant. Manufactured in the liver, squalene is a precursor for cholesterol, the fat that is the essential building block for hormones and part of the surface of all cells. It is also found in a variety of foods, including eggs and olive oil, over-the-counter medications, and health supplements. Squalene can be purchased at health food stores in its more commonly known form, "shark liver oil."

In the early 1970s, UCLA Medical Center scientist Carl M. Pearson began experimenting with a variety of edible oils, hoping to discover a safer, less toxic vaccine adjuvant. His assumption was that because these oils were naturally occurring and could be metabolized by the body they would be safe.

In his well-chronicled book, *Vaccine A: The Government Experiment That's Killing Our Soldiers and Why GIs Are Only The First Victims*, award-winning investigative journalist, Gary Matsumoto, gives an excellent explanation of the difference between *ingesting* an edible compound and *injecting* one into the body:

> "Intuitively, this premise seems somewhat dubious: Your body could metabolize a cheeseburger, for instance, but you couldn't liquefy it in a blender and inject the resulting slurry [into your arm], and then expect to feel well in the morning."[21]

The same holds true for squalene in shark liver oil and other edible oils. Research was conducted throughout the 1980s and 1990s using metabolizable oils, hoping to find an adjuvant to use in vaccines that didn't induce an antibody response. Many different oils were tried before Chiron settled on MF59, an adjuvant composed of squalene and two emulsifying agents, called Tween80 and Span®85. Mixed together, these compounds form an oil-in-water emulsion with uniform droplets less than one micron in diameter. The description on the patent application for MF59 states:

> "Any metabolizable oil, particularly from an animal, fish or vegetable source, may be used herein. It is essential that the oil be metabolized by the host to which it is administered, otherwise the oil component may cause abscesses, granulomas or *even carcinomas*, or (when used in veterinary practice) may make the meat of vaccinated birds and animals unacceptable for human consumption due to the deleterious effect the unmetabolized oil may have on the consumer."
> [Emphasis added.][22]

Scientific data, published in peer-reviewed journals, show that injected squalene is not metabolized like a food passing through the intestinal tract. Injected squalene droplets in vaccine research are considered to be "metabolized" when immune cells interact with them, transport them through the lymphatic system, and form antibodies to them. In other words, if squalene molecules remain in tissues (unmetabolized), toxic reactions can occur.

Pearson and his associates at UCLA injected dozens of oils, including squalene, into rats and found that *all* the oils were toxic, inducing arthritis with varying degrees of severity. Based on their ability to cause arthritis, the oils were assigned "arthritis scores," ranging from (+), considered to be mildly toxic, to (++++), which was "guaranteed to cripple." Squalene was given a score of (+++). In addition, *all* rats injected with squalene developed an MS-like disease that left them crippled, dragging their paralyzed hindquarters across their cages.[23]

Similarly, when molecules of squalene are injected into humans, even at concentrations as small as 10 to 20 parts per billion, the oil can lead to self-destructive immune responses, such as autoimmune arthritis and lupus.[24]

Several mechanisms have been proposed to explain this reaction. Metabolically, squalene stimulates an immune response excessively and nonspecifically. More than two dozen peer-reviewed scientific papers from ten different laboratories throughout the U.S., Europe, Asia, and Australia have been published documenting the development of autoimmune disease in animals injected with squalene-based adjuvants. A convincing proposal for why this occurs can be explained through the concept of "molecular mimicry" in which an antibody created against the squalene in MF59 can cross-react with the body's squalene on the surface of human cells. The destruction of the body's squalene can lead to debilitating autoimmune and central nervous system diseases.

The squalene in MF59 is not the only cause for concern. One of its components, Tween80 (polysorbate 80), is considered to be inert but is far from it. A study in December 2005 discovered that Tween80 can cause anaphylaxis, a potentially fatal reaction characterized by a sharp drop in blood pressure, hives, and breathing difficulties.

Researchers concluded that the severe reaction was not a typical allergic response characterized by the combination of IgE antibodies and the release of histamines; it was caused by a serious disruption that had occurred within the immune system.[25, 26]

MF59 and similar adjuvants are capable of accelerated activation of the immune system, particularly the innate (inborn) or cell-mediated immune system. Once the immune reaction is "turned on," there is no "switch" to turn it off. The long-term reactions are unknown and most likely will not be known. Following patients for an extended period to look for the development of serious reactions is not what the vaccine industry is interested in studying.

Vaccine clinical trials are aimed primarily at two results: 1) the assessment of reactions, usually within five to 14 days, of receiving the vaccine, and 2) the development of an "adequate antibody response." If the numbers of reactions are acceptably low and the antibody level in the blood is found to be acceptably high, the vaccine is considered to be safe and effective.

But there are problems with this conclusion. For one, it can take longer than 14 days to develop an autoimmune reaction in the body; in fact, it can take months.

> Pediatric vaccines that contain polysorbate 80 (Tween80) are:
>
> DTaP (Infanrix)
> DTaP (Tripedia)
> DTaP+Hib (TriHib)
> DTaP+HepB+IPV (Pediarix)
> Hepatitis A/Hepatitis B (Twinrix)

No long-term studies have been designed to investigate the development of these problems because these studies are expensive and time-consuming. Manufacturers conclude that the number of severe reactions are so small that they are not statistically significant, deeming them not worthy of study. And of course the FDA and IOM have the prerogative of declaring that "no causal relationship exists," even if the studies were undertaken by independent investigators.

The second problem is the definition of "effectiveness" used by clinical investigators. Most clinicians interpret effective to mean protective. In other words, if a vaccine is declared effective the person who receives it will be protected from infection. However, in vaccine research, effectiveness is defined as the vaccine's ability to induce an acceptably high antibody response, called a titer. The assumption is made that if the titer is elevated, protection is automatically conferred. This cornerstone argument supporting the use of vaccines has not been proven. In fact, the medical journal *Vaccine* published an article in 2001, clearly stating, "It is known that, in many instances, antigen-specific *antibody titers do not correlate with protection.*" [Emphasis added.][27] This means you can get the vaccine, develop antibodies, and *still* get the disease the vaccine was designed to protect you from. In addition, you get all the risks that come with the toxic vaccine components.

In spite of the known risks, MF59 was licensed for use by Chiron in 1997 to be used in its European influenza vaccine, Fluad®. The new adjuvant was chosen over concerns that aluminum did not substantially increase the antibody level in elderly patients who received a flu shot, but when MF59 was added, the antibody response more than doubled. The vaccine was deemed "safe and effective" by the investigators, but the results of the study could be seriously flawed. The clinical trial involved only elderly people in nursing homes; the average age was 71.5 years. If autoimmune problems such as fatigue and joint pain developed in this geriatric population, doctors might attribute these complaints only to old age.[28] If autoimmune problems occur in the general population after vaccination, doctors may well attribute these complaints to *anything but the vaccine.*

If the term MF59 rings a bell, it may be through its association with the anthrax vaccine. Gary Matsumoto's book, *Vaccine A* is a bone-chilling account of MF59 used in the anthrax vaccine given to tens of thousands of U.S troops going to the Gulf. This squalene-containing, unlicensed, experimental vaccine has been implicated as the cause of Gulf War Syndrome in thousands of military men and women.

Even though several clinical trials are currently underway to test a variety of squalene-based adjuvants, it appears likely that at least one of the pandemic vaccines will contain MF59. The warning given by Matsumoto in his book regarding the widespread use of MF59 is sobering: "The unethical experiments detailed in [my] book are ongoing, with little prospect of being self-limiting because they have been shielded from scrutiny and public accountability by national security concerns." He was referring to the anthrax vaccine and the military. However, because squalene-containing adjuvants could be a key ingredient in a whole new generation of vaccines intended for mass immunization around the globe, the problems may be just over the horizon.

The grave reality is that despite denials from the government, the vaccine industry, and the military, the highly-recommended book, *Vaccine A,* is a premonition of the serious health problems to come when MF59 or similar adjuvants are used in vaccines for the general population.

Additional studies are underway to evaluate the use of MF59 to create a "more effective" influenza vaccine. MF59, first used in 1997 after the avian flu outbreak in Hong Kong, has been shown in clinical trials to increase the response to viruses by allowing the use of a lower-than-normal amount of viral antigen. By adding MF59, 89 percent of the recipients developed a high level of antibodies after just one injection of the 1997 flu shot.[29]

In a press release issued on October 28, 2005, Chiron announced that by using its "highly immunogenic" adjuvant the smallest possible dose of viral antigen—3.75 micrograms, which is one-fourth the dose used in seasonal influenza vaccine—could be used. This makes MF59 a current front-runner of all other adjuvant candidates for inclusion in the pandemic vaccine.[30]

In 1997, a website was established on the Internet by Dr. Stephen Barrett called "Quackwatch." Its mission statement was "to combat health-related frauds, myths, fads, and fallacies."

Over the years, practitioners of alternative and integrative medicine have been mercilessly attacked by this self-proclaimed "protector of society" for everything from the use of vitamins and supplements to advocating acupuncture. This was done under the guise of "investigating questionable claims, answering inquiries about products and services, reporting illegal marketing, and attacking misleading advertising on the Internet." The careers of many honest, hard-working doctors who were practicing sensible, non-drug-based medicine—and helping people to get well—have been seriously damaged personally and professionally by the accusations of "Quackwatch."

Now, imagine this scenario: A practitioner of alternative medicine proclaims he has found a way to protect people from infectious diseases. He has created a suspension containing multiple viruses combined with a variety of potentially cancer-causing cells that originated from monkey and dog kidneys, caterpillar eggs, and retina cells from aborted human fetuses. Into the mix he has added formaldehyde, aluminum, mercury, a variety of other toxic chemicals called "preservatives," and an adjuvant made from shark liver oil—known to cause autoimmune diseases—called squalene. Proclaimed as a "wonder drug," the injectable potion is marketed for use by everyone in the world. Most importantly, the slurry is targeted for use in babies with injections starting at two months of age.

What would state medical boards, the FDA, and the U.S. government do to this "alternative" practitioner? He would be declared a heretic (maybe a lunatic). He would be dragged into court, be prosecuted, and have his license to practice medicine revoked. Depending on what had happened to the innocents who believed his rhetoric, he might be tried for malpractice, or worse, charged with murder.

Knowing what is in the flu shot, how it is made, and its potential cancer-causing ramifications, why aren't the companies that make them and the doctors who administer them held liable for producing a "quack therapy"? Recall Dr. Heneine's observations at the CBER meeting–that "specific pathogen-free" specimens are not the same as "pathogen-free." Knowing what's in those eggs—and what's coming through that needle—is very important to your life, especially since recent studies have pointed out serious concerns. The flu shot has not been proven safe, and it isn't nearly as effective as proponents want us to believe.

Chapter 10: Mandatory Vaccination: Is It Possible?

Starting points:
- President Bush proposes Project BioShield I
- Senator Frist gets it done for Pharma
- Liability for the vaccine industry not needed: It's been around for 20 years
- Executive orders and mandatory vaccination

Until recently, the concept of mandatory mass vaccination has been only a worrisome far-off possibility. Vaccination laws are passed and monitored at the state level, not mandated or enforced at the federal level. But the groundwork to change all that began three years ago on January 28, 2003, during President George W. Bush's State of the Union Address. On that fateful night, Bush revealed the creation of Project BioShield, a comprehensive effort to develop and make available modern, effective drugs and vaccines to protect against attack by biological and chemical weapons. The initial stage of the program was estimated to cost $5.6 billion over ten years.

Project BioShield set forth three major initiatives: 1) creating a permanent "indefinite funding authority" to spur development of medical countermeasures enabling the government to "purchase vaccines and other therapies as soon as experts believe that they can be made safe and effective," 2) conferring new authority to the NIH to speed research and development of drugs and vaccines that would counter bioterrorism threats, and 3) authorizing emergency fast track provisions for the release of treatments—drugs and vaccines—still waiting for approval by the FDA "in the event of an emergency."[1]

As sweeping as the provisions seemed to be, the legislation failed to include key provisions sought by the drug companies— complete liability protection for all its bioterrorism products. Many bills were introduced for this purpose by both the House and the Senate throughout 2003, 2004, and 2005–13 bills in 2005 alone–in an attempt to secure protection for the industry through federal law. It wasn't until October 17, 2005, when the Biodefense and Pandemic Vaccine and Drug Development Act of 2005 (known as BioShield II) put the pledge to "make good" for drug makers on the front burner.

Introduced by senators Bill Frist (R-TN) and Richard Burr (R-NC), the bill was accelerated through the Senate Health, Education, Labor, and Pensions (HELP) Committee, without hearings. Its purpose, according to Burr's news release, was to create a partnership between the government and private corporations that would "rapidly develop effective drugs and vaccines to protect the United States from deliberate, accidental, and natural incidents involving biological pathogens."[2]

The introduction of BioShield II raised the stakes to a new level. Named S.1873, the legislation was designed to give unprecedented advantages to the industry and remove or severely weaken all of the safeguards preventing dangerous vaccines, drugs, and medical devices from reaching consumers.[3]

Public outrage began almost immediately. While web sites, news outlets, and nationwide radio hosts began to decry the unbelievable benefits that passage of this bill would convey to the drug companies, dozens of activist groups representing thousands of constituents rallied a campaign to notify Congress of their dissatisfaction with S.1873. Faxes, emails, and phone calls conveyed message after message opposing the carte blanche promises about to be handed to the drug makers. Because the outcry against S.1873 was so strong, the possibility of its passage appeared to be remote.

To circumvent this public outrage, Senate Majority Leader Bill Frist attached a shortened version of the bill to the 2006 Department of Defense Appropriations Bill, HR 2863, *literally* at the eleventh hour, giving sweeping, unprecedented immunity for drug companies. Called "Division E—Public Readiness and Emergency Preparedness Act," Frist's addendum added 40 pages to an existing 423-page bill at 11:20 on Saturday night, December 17, 2005, well after the House Appropriation Committee members had reached final agreement on the defense bill, and signed off, and most had gone home.

Appalled, Representative Dave Obey (D-WI), ranking member of the House Appropriations Committee, made the following statement on the floor of the House on December 22, 2005:

> "When the president requested $7 billion to begin a much belated crash program to develop a new generation of vaccines and antiviral drugs to combat a potential flu pandemic, the Republican majority responded by cutting [that request] in half. When I asked Senator Ted Stevens (R-AK) in conference why we shouldn't fund the rest of the administration's request...he responded that because liability protection language for manufacturers had not been adopted, long-range funding should be withheld.
>
> "The Conference Committee [on the Defense Appropriations Bill] ended its work with an understanding, both verbal and in writing, that there would be no—*I repeat no*—legislative liability protection language inserted in this bill. And because the Republican Majority told us *it did not want any compensation program for victims* to come out of the discretionary portion of the budget, no funding was provided for that either.
>
> "But after the [committee] finished at 6 p.m., Senator Frist marched over to the House side of the Capitol, about four hours later, and insisted 40 pages of legislation—which I have in my hand—40 pages of

legislation that had never been seen by conferees, be attached to the bill.

"Speaker [Dennis Hastert R-IL] joined Frist's insistence, and without a vote of the conferees, the legislation was unilaterally and arrogantly inserted into the bill, after the conference was over. [This was] a blatantly abusive power play by two of the most powerful men in Congress.

"We then discovered that this language provided all sorts of insulation for pharmaceutical companies, and that this insulation applied not just to drugs developed to deal with the [avian] flu, but in fact applied to a far broader range of products."

After itemizing the problems associated with the "Division E" language, Representative Obey went on to say:

"Mr. Speaker, the Committee system was created years ago to protect the public interest, so legislation would be carefully reviewed before it was placed before the body for consideration. But that protection was arbitrarily by-passed by the Leadership in both Houses.

"This is the second time that this Congress has supinely done the bidding of the pharmaceutical industry in the dead of night. The first time, a vote was held open for three hours while the Republican Majority twisted arms to create the complex and ridiculously confusing prescription drug bill that our seniors are now so desperately trying to understand—a bill that was *ushered through this institution by over 600 lobbyists* and that protected [drug] companies by preventing the government from even attempting to negotiate lower drug prices.

"If I thought that denying unanimous consent on this bill would force the Majority to eliminate that language, I would object. *But, Mr. Speaker, it has also been made quite clear to me that the Majority will not relent on the language that insulates drug companies.* [Emphasis added.]

"So Mr. Speaker, I want it to be clear that the action to insert this special interest language in the bill is in my view a corruption of the legislative practices of the House. When Congress returns in January, I intend to raise a question about the privileges of the House, highlighted by this action, because it has brought discredit to the House and should disturb every Member who serves here.

"No Member of Congress, no matter how powerful, should be able to unilaterally insist that provisions that were never discussed and never debated in the Conference should be slipped in to that Conference report without a vote of that same Conference.

"This is what happens when there are no checks and balances, when one party controls the White House, the Senate, and the House and respects no limits on its own use of power. We have been placed in this position because the House Republican Leadership has sent Members home for the Christmas holidays with the message to the Senate that we would not be here [to review changes made by the Senate]. That was irresponsible and the country will pay the price. This institution will pay a price as well, in terms of diminished respect from the people we were elected to represent. Members on both sides know it, and it is time to have a modicum of respect for the way we do the people's business.

"This is a shameful and shabby way to end the worst session of Congress I've experienced in 36 years in Congress. I most reluctantly withdraw my reservation because lodging an objection at this point would simply delay the shameful inevitable."[4]

The nefarious language that Congressman Obey was objecting to in the "Division E" addendum deserves every bit of his tirade. Senator Ted Kennedy (D-MA) commented, "Generally around here we measure who the winners are and who the losers are, and we have seen over the period of the last year, year-and-a-half, how the drug companies come out [winners] time and time again, but never, never, ever, ever like they have with this sweetheart deal."[5]

Senator Frist (a medical doctor) handed the drug companies (a special interest group) more immunity than any bill that has ever been passed by Congress. The legislation provides at least four sweeping provisions:

1. Immunity from liability for *all* drugs, vaccines, or biological products deemed as a "covered countermeasure" in the event of an outbreak of any kind. The proposal is not in any way limited to only new drugs or vaccines developed under the umbrella of "bioterrorism" or "pandemic" protection. The proposal is so broad that it could include drugs like Tylenol®, Advil®...and would have applied to Vioxx®.

2. Immunity for *any* product used for *any* public health emergency declared by the secretary of HHS. As explained below, the authority to declare an emergency now rests completely in the hands of the secretary of HHS—*an appointed, non-medical person who has no accountability to the general public*. The president's person, hand-picked to be part of his inner circle, will have the power to mandate that vaccines and other medications be given to the American people.

3. Immunity from accountability, no matter what a drug company did wrong. Even if the company's dirty facility created a batch of contaminated vaccines that resulted in death or injury to thousands of people, the drug company will not be held accountable.

4. Immunity from law suits. A person who suffers any type of loss will be legally prohibited from suing the drug companies; they now have immunity from almost everything, perhaps even murder. The bill provisions provide a mechanism for filing a lawsuit, but the language explicitly prevents frivolous suits by setting a standard for liability more rigid than any known standard of negligence. According to the American Trial Lawyers Association, the bill contains language never before seen in any proposal. In simple

terms, if a claim is filed by a plaintiff it can go forward only if the injured party *can prove* that the company performed an act of "willful misconduct" that resulted in an injury or a death. In other words, the injured party would have to prove the vaccine maker intentionally caused them harm. Unbelievably, *even then* the drug company is still immune from accountability. Even if a pharmaceutical company *knowingly harms people,* the company will be immune from legal prosecution unless the U.S. attorney general initiates "enforcement action" against the drug company in the name of the claimant. This means the U.S. government would have to go to bat for the plaintiff against the drug company for the lawsuit to move forward.

Keep in mind that the person who rammed this bill through to completion is a medical doctor who at one time took an oath to "do no harm."[6]

Liability protection not needed

Senator Frist wasn't acting alone in his zeal for drug company protection. The push to pass this protective legislation was actually started by the Bush administration. At a press conference held November 1, 2005, President Bush urged increased financial benefits for the drug companies and "relief from the burden of litigation" for the vaccine manufacturers, stating:

> "I'm also asking Congress to remove one of the greatest obstacles to domestic vaccine production: *the growing burden of litigation.* In the past three decades, the number of vaccine manufacturers in America has plummeted, as the industry has been flooded with lawsuits. Today, there is only one manufacturer in the United States that can produce influenza vaccine. That leaves our nation vulnerable in the event of a pandemic. We must increase the number of vaccine manufacturers in our country and improve our domestic production capacity. *So Congress must pass liability protection for the makers of life-saving vaccines."* [Emphasis added.][7]

President Bush and his advisors should be held accountable for yet another set of misinformation propagated to the under-informed general public. A recent study in the *Journal of the American Medical Association* found there had been only 10 lawsuits in the last 20 years over flu vaccines. This surprisingly low number led the authors to conclude that drug companies withdrew from the vaccine business mainly because of low-profit margins and unpredictable demand, not over liability concerns.[8] Moreover, protective legislation for the vaccine industry has been in place for nearly 20 years.

In the 1980s, drug companies were opting out of the vaccine business, ostensibly due to skyrocketing legal costs needed to defend lawsuits filed for vaccine injuries. By convincing government officials that the National Vaccine Program was the cornerstone of the U.S. public health policy, President Reagan was strong-armed into signing into law the Childhood Vaccine Injury Act of 1986, a law to protect drug manufacturers from lawsuits arising out of injuries caused by childhood vaccines. Part of that legislation included the National Vaccine Injury Compensation Program (NVICP), a mechanism for injured parties to recover damages from harm caused by vaccines.[9]

The intent of the NVICP was to create an alternative to civil litigation, meaning that if an injury occurred due to a vaccine, negligence would not have to be proven and compensation would be automatically paid by the government for the "personal sacrifice" that had been made by that individual—agreeing to be vaccinated for the "good of the whole." The legislation was modeled after the compensation portion of the Swine Flu Act. As straightforward as it seems—or as it was intended to be—there are serious flaws in the program.

The most glaring issue is that only certain vaccine injuries are eligible for compensation. The government has created a list referred to as the "Vaccine Injury Compensation Table," or simply "The Table," detailing the specific injuries or conditions that must be met for a person *to be eligible* for compensation. In other words, sustaining an injury doesn't automatically trigger compensation. The Table contains the legal definitions of the medical conditions allowed as statutory "presumption of causation." Simply put, the definitions in The Table determine whether or not an injury was actually caused by the vaccine. Not the doctor who cared for the person; not a person who experienced or witnessed the event. The "diagnosis" of a vaccine injury is made by a table created by politicians and medicobureaucrats at the CDC.

The definitions in The Table go beyond setting the definitions of a vaccine injury. The Table clearly defines the *time frame in which the injury must occur* to qualify for government compensation. If the alleged injury and time sequence do not match those in The Table, the "burden of proof" is placed on the injured party, meaning, the person must go up against the government and the pharmaceutical industry to prove that the vaccine caused the injury. Obviously, with the deck stacked against the injured, compensation for damages is nearly always denied.[10]

For example, an "allowable definition" for reaction caused by the DTaP vaccine is anaphylactic shock. According to The Table, the time interval for this injury to manifest must be no more than four hours after the vaccine was given. If a child develops anaphylaxis, say, 10 hours or more after receiving the shot, it is considered to be "off The Table," and by the government's definition, the anaphylaxis was not caused by the vaccine. In this scenario, the parent would not be eligible for compensation, and the only remaining recourse would be to pursue damages through civil court, a long, arduous process with little hope of winning.

Another example is injury caused by the hepatitis B vaccine, which was added to the Compensation Table in 1997. Only one event is eligible for government compensation: anaphylaxis, or death from anaphylaxis, which must occur within four hours of receiving the vaccine. Despite the fact that medical literature is replete with case reports of autoimmune and neurological dysfunction following hepatitis B vaccination in both children and adults, anaphylaxis is the only injury that qualifies for compensation. All other complications are considered to be a "coincidence" and not caused by the vaccine.

These are but two examples of the thousands of serious side effects reported after vaccination to the Vaccine Adverse Events Reporting System (VAERS, part of the NVICP). These reports can be filed electronically by a parent, a doctor, or any concerned party. VAERS reports are the chronicle of events observed to be caused by vaccines, but most researchers, including the CDC, view the reports as merely points of interest. The CDC and the drug companies claim that vaccine injuries are "rare," occurring in no more than one or two persons per million shots given. If The Table is used as the measure for the number of reactions, that is an accurate statement. There are relatively few cases of anaphylaxis and immediate deaths following vaccines. However, if all reactions are considered, including those published in and supported by the medical literature, the actual number of injuries associated with vaccines is staggering.

Between 11,000 to 12,000 reports of vaccine reactions are filed with VAERS each year. Of these, 15 percent are considered "serious" (i.e., necessitating a trip to the emergency room, requiring a hospitalization, or resulting in a permanent disability). However, most people—even most doctors—aren't aware of the VAERS system, and underreporting is a substantial problem. Overall, it is estimated that less than 1 percent of all adverse events from drugs and vaccines are reported.[11] Based on these estimates, there could actually be up to 1.2 million vaccine-related adverse events occurring *every year* in America, a truly jolting number.

Language written into the NVICP Act granted the secretary of HHS broad discretionary authority to alter The Table. The *intent* was to introduce flexibility into the system by allowing the list of conditions on The Table to expand and be more inclusive as additional injuries became apparent. Because an increasing number of vaccines were under development, it was assumed that additional injuries would be identified at some point in the future that would require compensation. However, the exact opposite came to pass. Former Secretary Donna Shalala used her discretionary authority to *remove* compensable events from The Table and redefine permanent injuries, placing an even greater burden upon petitioners to prove that vaccination caused an injury or a death.

While patients struggle with massive medical and legal bills attempting to receive compensation for damages through Vaccine Court, salaried government administrators, seasoned trial lawyers, court officials, and their administrative staffs are paid with public funds throughout the compensation process, fighting against the citizens and their attorneys who are less likely to take on vaccine injury cases due to these bureaucratic and political hurdles.[12] The drug companies protect their product by paying tens of thousands of dollars to "expert witnesses"—physicians and scientists—to testify, using their credentials to disprove the claims initiated by parents. Even with years of hard work, the number of claims that actually receive compensation is about one out of seven, or less than 15 percent.[13]

A vaccine gains liability protection when it is approved by the Advisory Committee for Immunization Practices (ACIP) and added as a requirement to the routine pediatric vaccination schedule. Once approved for babies, the vaccine has an immediate market share (there are approximately 77,000 live births per week in this country), and the government, the manufacturer, and the doctor or nurse who administers the vaccine all have automatic protection from lawsuits. As stated by Paul A. Offit, MD, chief of the division of infectious diseases at Children's Hospital of Philadelphia, the NVICP is basically a way "to protect pharmaceutical companies from ambushes by the tort system."[14] It appears that the priority of the U.S. government and the U.S. Public Health Service has long been to protect drug companies from overcompensating families for injuries—including deaths—resulting from vaccination.

With the passage of Frist's addendum, drug companies have been handed a whole new level of unparalleled liability protection. Severe side effects from vaccines and drugs will no doubt occur, because there is no incentive to ensure safety without the pressure of liability. In addition, vaccine injuries increase product sales—if a person is injured, more drugs are necessary to treat the injury.

In a post-9/11 era, bioterrorism products can be "fast-tracked" and not put through the same lengthy approval process as other drugs and vaccines. In addition, they won't have to go through the arduous process of first becoming pediatric mandates to be protected. Any drug or vaccine declared to be part of the War on Terror will get preferential treatment and huge financial benefits.

Almost before the ink had dried on Frist's addendum, it was announced on December 22, 2005, that Fluarix® would be the first vaccine to receive FDA accelerated approval for use in the U.S. Touted as an "effective government/industry collaboration to bolster the flu vaccine supply," Fluarix (approved in 1998 for use in other countries, but never tested or licensed for use in the U.S.) was fast-tracked for the 2005-2006 flu season.[15] The FDA based the accelerated approval on four clinical studies done in Europe involving approximately 1,200 adults. FDA Commissioner Lester Crawford crowed that the "accelerated approval has allowed us to evaluate and approve Fluarix in record time."

NIAID Director, Anthony Fauci, MD, added, "This effort is a model for the type of effective collaboration that will be needed to produce vaccines in the event of an influenza pandemic." Definitely a sign of things to come.

The groundwork has been laid for mandatory vaccination

Using quarantines as a disease-prevention tool began during the fourteenth century in an effort to protect coastal cities from plague epidemics. Ships arriving from infected ports were required to sit at anchor for 40 days before landing. Therefore, the practice of quarantine acquired its name from the Italian words *quaranta giorni,* which means "40 days."[16]

In 1944, with the passage of the Public Health Service Act (USPHSA), the federal government's authority to quarantine was clearly established for the first time. In 1953, the Public Health Service became part of the Department of Health, Education, and Welfare (HEW), which later morphed into the Department of Health and Human Services (HHS). In 1967, the role of quarantine was transferred to the National Communicable Disease Center, now known as the CDC.

About the same time as the establishment of the USPHS (1946), a list of communicable diseases that could be corralled using quarantines was declared through Executive Order (E.O.) 9708, issued by President Truman. Periodically updated over the last 50 years, the list explicitly includes the following infections: cholera, diphtheria, infectious tuberculosis, plague (typhoid), smallpox, yellow fever, and viral hemorrhagic fevers (such as Lassa, Marburg, Ebola, Crimean-Congo, and South American).

On April 4, 2003, President Bush added SARS to the list of communicable diseases that could be quarantined by signing Executive Order 13295. SARS is described as "a disease associated with fever and signs and symptoms of pneumonia or other respiratory illness. It is transmitted from person to person predominantly by the aerosolized or droplet route, and if spread in the population would have severe public health consequences."[18] At the urging of the CDC, this description was kept intentionally vague. The language opens the potential for detaining mild to moderately ill persons completely against their will.[18]

Title 42 of the Public Health Service Act has many subsections. The regulations contained in Chapter 6A, Section G, called "Quarantine and Inspection," give the Public Health Service full responsibility for preventing the transmission of communicable diseases. Prior to 2002, the steps were clearly defined. On the recommendation of a *consensus* of the National Advisory Health Committee and in *agreement with* the surgeon general, the president would be notified of a disease thought to cause significant risk to the general population. The name of that disease would be added to the list of risky communicable diseases by a presidential Executive Order. However, this chain of command was changed with the passage of the "Public Health Security and Bioterrorism Preparedness and Response Act of 2002," also referred to as "The Bioterrorism Act."

Section 142 of the Bioterrorism Act was rewritten to "streamline and clarify" previously established provisions regarding quarantine. Now, only two opinions—instead of a consensus of the National Advisory Committee—are needed to decide whether a disease warrants quarantine: the opinions of the secretary of HHS and the surgeon general.[19] In the original provisions the surgeon general made the decisions *in consultation with* the president and the secretary of HHS. With the passage of the Bioterrorism Act, decisions are now made by the secretary of HHS *"in consultation with the surgeon general."* This is an important distinction. The surgeon general is a medical doctor; the secretary of

115

HHS is a politician. Notably, both officials are *appointees* and completely removed from accountability to the general public. Quite frankly, they have been handed enormous power over the citizens of this country.

One of the most unnerving changes in The Bioterrorism Act of 2002 is the new definition of who can be detained. Previously, only those "reasonably thought to be infected" were to be quarantined. In the revised act, a person can be mandatorily confined if he or she is in a *"pre-communicable stage,"* meaning the disease *"would be likely to cause a public health emergency* if transmitted to other individuals." [Emphasis added.][20]

Executive Order 13295, signed in 2003, further secured the decision-making power regarding who could be quarantined directly to the secretary of HHS. Beyond simply adding SARS to the list of communicable illnesses, the E.O. explicitly states that the secretary, *"at his discretion,"* can determine whether a particular infectious disease is serious enough to arrange for the apprehension and examination of persons "reasonably believed to be infected."

The combined effect of the Bioterrorism Act of 2002 and E.O. 13295 is that the secretary of HHS can issue a directive for a person to be quarantined under the "suspicion" of exposure or "possibility" that he or she *may* become sick. A cough or sneezing from seasonal allergies could put a person at risk of being quarantined without recourse and for an extended period. Penalties for violating the quarantine order "without permission of the quarantine officer in charge" can be a fine of "up to $1,000 and/or imprisonment for up to one year."[21]

That's a lot of power.

Keep in mind: Apprehension could theoretically occur for something as benign as bronchitis, a respiratory infection that has "signs and symptoms of pneumonia."

All of these mechanisms—Bioterrorism laws enhancing the mechanism for mandatory quarantines, Executive Orders, and power given exclusively to the secretary of HHS—were in place *before* the H5N1 outbreaks started in 2004. Then on April 1, 2005, President Bush added "influenza caused by novel or re-emergent influenza viruses that are causing, or have the potential to cause, a pandemic" to the list of quarantinable diseases through an amendment to E.O. 13295.[22]

Buried near the end of the Division E Amendment, tacked on by Senator Frist, is language alluding to the ominous situation in which mandatory vaccination could indeed occur by order of the secretary of HHS, without exception, and the overriding of state exemption laws.

Section (b)(1) of Division-E states that, if the secretary makes a determination that a "disease, health condition, or threat" constitutes a public health emergency, the secretary may make a declaration and then recommend "the *administration, or use of one or more covered countermeasures."* A covered countermeasure is defined as a "pandemic product, *vaccine* or drug."

Section (b)(7) of Division-E states that no federal or state court will have jurisdiction to review any action taken by the secretary. His ruling will *preempt any and all state laws* that are different from or in conflict with his declaration." The distinct lack of checks and balances undeniably puts the public at risk and is indeed frightening. It appears that an appointed politician has been handed the power to order vaccination for everyone.

Near the end of Division-E, participants are assured that the plan "to administer or use a covered countermeasure" will include education with respect to contraindications, and mentions briefly that the vaccination program is "voluntary." Will the media make everyone aware of the one-line provision that ensures the right to refuse? A quote by U.S. Representative Ron Paul (R-TX) says it all: "When we give government the power to make medical decisions for us, we, in essence, accept that the state owns our bodies."[23]

It appears the government is ramping up for mass vaccination, and possibly mandatory vaccination. The "trial run" occurred in 2002 when funding for mass vaccination clinics and vaccination drills were approved during the smallpox concern. The vaccination clinics never materialized, but just like community-wide disaster drills, lessons were learned for future use.

Mandated at a high level

The pressure to pass protective legislation for the benefit of drug companies didn't just come from drug company lobbyists. There is a worldwide plan being developed for global vaccination that includes protection for manufacturers of bioterrorism drugs and vaccines. From the WHO to local newspapers, many entities are disseminating the same message. At a global meeting held at the WHO in November 2005, the director general of the WHO was quoted as saying, "It is only a matter of time before an avian flu virus—most likely H5N1— acquires the ability to be transmitted from human to human, sparking the outbreak of human pandemic influenza. We don't know when this will happen. *But we do know that it will happen.*" [Emphasis added.][24] That's a really strong statement. Stating emphatically that it "will happen" sounds as if they know something we don't know, and the outcome has been predetermined.

First published in 1999, the WHO Global Pandemic Planning document demonstrates that preparedness meetings have been ongoing for a long time—long before H5N1 outbreaks hit the world stage. Perhaps the U.S. Congress and the president are not operating independently in their urgency to protect the pharmaceutical industry and shuffle massive amounts of tax dollars into their already overflowing coffers.

The newest version of the WHO global planning document, released early in 2005, contains step-by-step guidelines of how human H5N1 infection will be handled at the international level *when* the pandemic arrives. The plan gives detailed instructions with objectives and action items to be followed at both the national and global levels. An examination of this plan makes it clear that the game plan from the WHO is being followed precisely by our government.

According to the WHO global plan, current conditions represent Phase 1, called the "Inter-Pandemic Period." The overarching goal during this period is to "strengthen influenza pandemic preparedness at the global, regional, national, and sub-national (local) levels." On page 27 of the document, Item Five gives the following instructions:

"Resolve liability and other legal issues linked to use of the pandemic vaccine for mass or targeted emergency vaccination campaigns, if not yet done."

This is a direct imperative from the WHO to governments, ordering them to absolve liability issues for the manufacturers of drugs, vaccines, and other products before the pandemic occurs. The mandate was important enough to give it a line item in the WHO's plan. And while none of the current documents come right out and say it, the intimations are very clear: Mass vaccinations, and even mandatory vaccination, are distinct possibilities *when* the pandemic hits and *when* the vaccine is available.

The following is summarized from the WHO document: "Pandemic Alert Period, Phase 5–Prevention and Containment."[25]

1. Implement interventions identified during contingency planning and new guidance provided by WHO.
2. Consider use of antivirals for early treatment of cases.
3. Assess efficacy and feasibility of prophylaxis for the purpose of attempting to contain outbreaks. *[This implies the use of Ring vaccination, a part of the smallpox containment plan.By definition, this means vaccinating all close contacts of the ill person. This has never been shown to be useful for containing influenza.]*
4. **Determine target population for vaccination;** if intervention agreed, implement as an emergency measure; assess impact. *[Emphasis added.]*
5. Consider deploying prototype pandemic vaccine, if available. *[This means that use of an unproven, marginally tested vaccine will be allowed.]*
6. If agreements are already in place with manufacturer(s), consider recommending cessation of seasonal vaccine production and initiation of full-scale pandemic vaccine production.
7. Adjust priority lists of persons to be vaccinated.
8. Plan for vaccine distribution and accelerate preparations for mass vaccination campaigns (e.g., education, legal/ liability issues) for when pandemic vaccine becomes available. [Emphasis added.]

It is undeniably clear that mass vaccination will be implemented. Whether or not the right to refuse will be retained remains to be seen.

Is there a mechanism for enforcement? The idea of National Guard troops or public health officials going door-to-door to forcibly vaccinate the entire population is difficult to imagine. The manpower and bureaucratic direction required for implementation of a program of that magnitude is lacking, and administrative issues would be a nightmare. However, broader enforcement tools are already in place and could easily be implemented to carry out mandatory vaccination.

For example, a "vaccine ID card" could be required for travel or to do business, and only those with a "government-authorized vaccine ID" would be allowed to move about the country—or the world. Another possibility is human microchips which has been under development for quite some time. The FDA approved an implantable, rice grain-sized microchip for use in humans in October 2004. The subcutaneously injected Radio Frequency Identification (RFID) chip, made by a company called VeriChip, is already gaining in popularity. VeriChip's biggest market is Mexico, where 18 members of the attorney general's staff were implanted with a chip to control access to a new government facility.[26] Other uses of the chip come to mind without overly stretching the imagination.

The young physician starts life with 20 drugs for each disease, and the old physician ends life with one drug for 20 diseases.
~Sir William Osler, Canadian Physician, 1849-1919

Chapter 11: The Scam of Tamiflu

Starting points:
- Neuraminidase inhibitors explained
- Relenza first to market; Tamiflu close behind
- Medical bust: It doesn't work
- Who benefits?

In addition to vaccines, two drugs considered to be covered countermeasures have been introduced to the market for the treatment and prevention of influenza. Observing that the ideal antiviral drug is effective against all types of influenza viruses, regardless of strain and irrespective of antigenic drifts and shifts, GlaxoWelcome seemed to meet that criteria when it developed Relenza®.

Recall that two prevalent protein antigens project from the surface of influenza viruses. One is called hemagglutinin (H), which plays a role in binding the cell receptors of the host, and the other is the enzyme neuraminidase (N), which plays an important role in the spread of viruses to other people. When a virus enters the host's cells, the (H) protein binds to a molecule called sialic acid, which sits on the surface of mucous cells. This lock-and-key configuration opens the door to the cell, allowing the virus to enter and start the process of self-replication.

After the new viral particles are formed within the cells of the host, they are released to find a new cell to invade. On the way out, the particle becomes coated with the sialic acid. If this coating remains intact, the covered (H) receptors cannot bind to a different cell. The virus has a self-cleaning solution: The neuraminidase enzyme (N) scrubs the molecules of sialic acid off the (H) binding sites. The clean (H) receptors on the newly formed viral particles are then ready to attach to the next cell. Without the work done by neuraminidase, (H) antigens would stay coated with sialic acid and the virus can't spread. It is through the discovery of this complex process that drugs known as neuraminidase inhibitors were developed, which work by disabling the action of the (N) enzyme.

Relenza: First to be released

On February 24, 1999, a special meeting of the Antiviral Drug Products Advisory Committee convened to discuss Relenza® (Zanamivir), a new product being accelerated into the market by GlaxoWelcome. Relenza is a powdered medication, delivered through an inhaler, developed for the treatment of uncomplicated flu caused specifically by influenza type A and type B infections. GlaxoWelcome's drug application to the FDA sought approval for use in adults and in adolescents at least 12 years of age.

Unusual in its scope, the Relenza application was quite different from those typically presented for consideration to the Advisory Committee. Debra Birnkrant, MD, from the FDA, opened the meeting by admitting that the committee usually discussed only drugs that were under consideration for treating "serious life-threatening diseases." Regarding Relenza, she went on to say:

> "This is a [drug] application for a disease which is acute and self-limited in the majority of patients, but could potentially infect the entire population and account for a substantial morbidity. This application was granted for a 'priority review' because influenza has the propensity to affect such a large portion of the population."

She closed her introduction by saying that reviewing the application was a way to keep HHS in the loop in order to prepare for an influenza pandemic.[1]

Given that it was a novel drug utilizing a unique delivery system, Relenza had encountered special difficulties during its clinical trials. A full day of testimonies and questions following her opening remarks brought several concerns to light.

The committee immediately raised concerns about the conflicting data GlaxoWelcome presented from its three clinical trials: one conducted in the United States and Canada, one in Europe, and one in the Southern Hemisphere. Of the 1,588 total subjects enrolled in the three studies, only 73 percent had culture-confirmed influenza. The rest—more than 25 percent of the study participants (428)—were included because they had "influenza-like" symptoms. That created a glaring but unaddressed problem with the sample selection: Relenza is effective only against influenza viruses and not other viruses that cause influenza-like illnesses. The committee agreed that participants who were not confirmed to be infected by an influenza A or B virus should not have been included in the trial.

The primary endpoint of the study involved measuring the "time to alleviation of symptoms," an arbitrary determination ranked on a diary card by the patient. Patients judged their symptoms as "none, mild, moderate, or severe" on a scale of zero to three with regard to fever, cough, headache, myalgia, and sore throat. To be considered "over the flu," patients needed to rank all symptoms as none or mild, and the patient's temperature had to be less than 100°F (37.8°C) for at least 24 hours.

The effectiveness of Relenza was dismal. All three trials showed inconsistent findings, with the largest of the three, the North American trial, demonstrating no effect at all. During both foreign trials, Relenza had only modest effectiveness. Nonetheless, GlaxoWelcome attempted to spin the results as a "smashing success," touting that symptoms had decreased by 2.5 days in the European trial and 1.5 days in the Southern Hemisphere trial. When the numbers were reworked by an FDA statistician, the results equated to a symptom-relief score of a meager 1.8 days in the first trial and a barely noticeable 1.1 days for the second.

The endpoint determination—based on the diary cards—troubled one of the conference attendees, Janet Wittes, PhD, a statistician and president of Statistics Collaborative, Inc. in Washington, D.C. She raised concerns about the subjective nature of the cards and questioned the validity of comparing the studies because the cards were distributed in different languages and in different countries. She asked, "I have a question about the diary cards in terms of the translations and the back translations. Given the subjective nature of those responses, how did you calibrate one language against another? How do we know that what one observes in one country is the same as in another? How do you know that the translation was perceived the same way across languages?"

Not missing a beat, GlaxoWelcome's representative, Dr. Michael Elliot, answered quickly: "We don't have a poll that measures perception. I think we just have to rest on our experience and assume that the translation is true to the meaning."[2] Given that the totals on the self-scored cards were the crucial determining factors for assessing the effectiveness of the medication, his answer was far from reassuring.

Further, the Advisory Committee was very apprehensive about the lack of data regarding the drug's use in high-risk patients, particularly those with preexisting lung conditions and heart disease. In the studies, "high risk" groups consisted of patients with asthma who averaged 37 years of age. James Stoller, PhD, head of the Respiratory Therapy Department in association with the Department of Pulmonary and Critical Care at the Cleveland Clinic, asked very specific questions about the use of "objective measurements" such as pulmonary function tests or peak flow values to determine the severity of the patient's lung disease.

Responding, Elliot admitted that objective measures were not used and that the severity of the participant's disease was based solely on the "opinion of the clinical investigator," largely determined by the number of medications the person was using. In other words, the more medications a person was on, the more severe the asthma was judged to be—another completely subjective judgement. Beyond that, the number of patients with severe lung disease (chronic obstructive pulmonary disease, or COPD), severe cardiac disease, or in the geriatric age group was "very small."[3] The committee had reason for serious concern over the paucity of data involving high-risk patients as they are the group targeted with drugs at the first sign of the flu.

In the end, the committee voted 14 to 3 *against approval* of the drug. One committee member, Dr. John Hamilton, professor of medicine from Duke University, remarked, "While I appreciate that every attempt was made to identify the endpoints, my impression of the data, especially from the North American study, is that there isn't sufficient efficacy to warrant me recommending this drug for my family or myself."[4]

Incredibly, despite concerns and lack of support by her own committee, Heidi M. Jolson, MD, MPH, director of the Division of Antiviral Drug Products at the FDA, proceeded to approve Relenza for use five months later. She defended her decision by saying, "I do not believe that the lack of a conclusive finding in the North American study negates the *robust demonstrations of efficacy* [emphasis added] in the European and Southern Hemisphere studies, particularly given the inherent difficulties in conducting trials for this indication. Overall, the totality of the data provides evidence that treatment with [Relenza] confers a modest reduction in time to alleviation of influenza symptoms."[5]

Even using GlaxoWelcome's statistics, rather than those arrived by the FDA statistician, the European trial decreased symptoms by 2.5 days, and the Southern Hemisphere trial decreased symptoms by 1.5 days over the placebo. By any measure this is hardly "robust efficacy."

Hence, Relenza became the first neuraminidase inhibitor to be marketed in the United States. Relenza was approved for adults and adolescents to be taken by intranasal spray twice daily for five days beginning within two days of the onset of symptoms. The big win for patients, at least from GlaxoWelcome's view, was that the drug could shorten symptoms by about one day when compared with doing nothing at all.[6]

One day. Again, hardly "robust efficacy."

No about face, just caution

The committee had justifiably raised concerns about the safety of Relenza in high-risk patients. Soon after the drug was approved, reports of serious complications started to role in as the first flu season was getting into full swing. A mere six months after approval, the FDA was forced to issue a Public Health Advisory highlighting problems with Relenza. Caution was advised concerning its use in patients with underlying asthma or chronic obstructive pulmonary disease (COPD), such as emphysema. The FDA received several reports of deteriorating lung function, ranging from bronchospasm (wheezing) to respiratory arrest (cessation of breathing), following the inhalation of Relenza in patients with chronic conditions. During that same flu season, from November 2, 1999, to June 30, 2000, the Canadian Adverse Drug Reaction Monitoring Program received 16 reports of suspected adverse reactions. Six were classified as "serious and unexpected," including one death.[7]

But instead of issuing a product recall, the FDA instead issued a warning with a recommendation to use "careful monitoring, proper observation, and appropriate supportive care, including the availability of short-acting bronchodialators," when prescribing this drug.[8] This begs the question: Why would the FDA recommend "careful monitoring" of a potentially life-threatening drug that relieves symptoms of the flu by only one day? In addition, why would any doctor be willing to prescribe it?

Tamiflu: Next on the market

Three months after the approval of Relenza, (October 1999) Tamiflu® (oseltamivir) became the first *oral* neuraminidase inhibitor approved by the FDA. Approval of the pill was based on the results of two double-blind trials conducted in 1997 and 1998 involving 1,358 patients. One trial was conducted in the United States, and the other involved patients from Canada, Europe, and Hong Kong. Only 62 percent had laboratory testing done, confirming influenza viruses as the cause of their symptoms. Like Relenza, Tamiflu is meant to inhibit the neuraminidase enzyme of influenza viruses; it has no effect against other microbes.

Similar to the Relenza trials, the effectiveness of the drug was judged by having participants complete self-assessment "symptom scores" to evaluate a reduction in influenza-associated symptoms. The "time to improvement of symptoms" was calculated from the time treatment started to the time when all symptoms (nasal congestion, sore throat, cough, aches, fatigue, headaches, and chills and sweats) decreased to none or mild. Despite the fact that symptom relief was only 1.3 days sooner with Tamiflu than for placebo, the FDA approved the drug for use.

It bears repeating that neuraminidase inhibitors work to block the (N) antigen of *influenza* viruses. They have no effect on other viruses that cause influenza-like illnesses. Amazingly enough, the drug gained approval after it was tested on *only 849 people* who were culture-confirmed influenza. In an FDA memorandum dated October 25, 1999, the director of the Division of Antiviral Drug Products, Heidi M. Jolson, MD, MPH, defended approval of the drug by saying:

> "The clinical relevance of the modest treatment benefit is a highly subjective question. It is my opinion that a one-day reduction in the duration of moderate-to-severe symptoms, including fever, is likely to be of clinical importance to many individuals.... Because influenza symptoms are self-limited in the majority of individuals, it is anticipated that many persons with influenza will neither require, nor desire treatment with antiviral medications."[9]

In addition to proposing Tamiflu for the treatment of influenza, two studies were submitted to the FDA in 1999 to gain approval for Tamiflu prevent the flu. In the first, published in the Journal of the American Medical Association (*JAMA*), 21 subjects were given either 100 or 200 milligrams of Tamiflu for 26 hours before being inoculated with influenza viruses. The control group, which consisted of only 12 people, were given a placebo prior to being inoculated with the virus. The results showed that eight of 12 people (66%), who were given the placebo, contracted the flu, while eight of 21 people (38%), who received Tamiflu, did not. This was lauded as a nearly 50 percent reduction in the incidence of the flu when Tamiflu is given as a preventative.[10] Considering that less than 100 patients were included in the trial, and an unequal number of participants were in each group, the success of the claim is significantly exaggerated.

At about the same time that the *JAMA* article was published, the results of a larger trial were announced in the *New England Journal of Medicine.* This study involved 1,559 healthy, non-vaccinated adults, who were randomized to receive either 75 milligrams of Tamiflu or 75 milligrams of a placebo, for six weeks during the peak of the influenza season. The incidence of the flu was only slightly less with Tamiflu, (1.2 percent) than with the placebo (4.8 percent), meaning that taking Tamiflu was barely more effective than doing nothing at all to prevent the flu.[11] Despite the trivial effectiveness reported in these two studies, the FDA approved the use of Tamiflu for the prevention of the flu.

The medical community plans to use Tamiflu to prevent the spread of viruses from an infected person to healthy persons. The most likely scenario for this recommendation will be toward nurses and other healthcare professionals working in hospital settings. The *JAMA* study reported that six of the 12 people who were given the placebo continued to shed the virus after they became ill. Conversely, viral shedding didn't occur at all among any of the

Using an aerosol machine, a treatment often used for asthma, can reduce the spread of viruses and bacteria. A small study involving 11 people found that some people exhale lager amounts of germs than others when they are sick. A six-minute aerosol treatment using saltwater demonstrated that the numbers of viruses or bacteria being exhaled was sharply reduced - by 72 percent - for up to six hours. Researchers concluded that, even though the study was small, the administration of a nebulized saline solution could dramatically reduce the spread of infection.

people who had taken Tamiflu. The claim that Tamiflu could stop the spread of flu viruses is based on the results of examining a scant 12 people with a claim of a 50% reduction in the number, (i.e. six of 12 compared to zero of 12).

Beyond the lackluster results for the treatment and prevention of influenza, nearly 10 percent of people who are prescribed Tamiflu can't tolerate the most common side effect—persistent nausea. With the course of treatment costing $100-$200 (depending on the dose used), perhaps the best course of action is to use aerosolized saline nasal spray which may be at least as effective and at minimal cost. [See insert.][12]

Stockpiling begins

On August 26, 2004, the HHS and the CDC released their draft of the "Pandemic Influenza Preparedness and Response Plan." In it, Tamiflu was highlighted as the antiviral drug to be stockpiled by the U.S. government and military as part of preparations for a possible influenza pandemic. Government models developed by two international research teams suggested a pandemic could be stopped if a "ring of contacts" around the first human cases were given Tamiflu to prevent the virus from infecting others. All the hype about the use of Tamiflu for treatment and prevention of influenza during the pandemic overlooked one egregious problem—there is no data regarding the effectiveness of Tamiflu for treating H5N1.

Even though Tamiflu is designed to inhibit the neuraminidase (N) enzyme of influenza viruses, it has been found to be more effective against some influenza subtypes than others. Recall that neuraminidase "scrubs" the sialic acid off the surface of the (H) receptor of a newly released virus. If the enzyme is inhibited, the cleansing "bath" doesn't occur, and the infection can't spread from cell to cell. If the drug works, it will stop the virus from spreading person-to-person.

In early screenings, Tamiflu was tested against all nine (N) subtypes. However, it is generally accepted among scientists that the pandemic strain—whether it is H5N1 or some other influenza virus—will contain surface antigen N1. In laboratory tests designed to evaluate Tamiflu's ability to inhibit the N1 neuraminidase, Tamiflu failed dismally. In order for it to work, *eight to 12 times* the recommended dose of the drug was needed to achieve the same level of inhibition as in other (N) subtypes.

When Tamiflu was tested specifically against H5N1 isolates from Vietnam and Thailand, an *additional* three-fold increase in the dose was required to stop the replication of the virus, meaning almost *30 times more Tamiflu* would be needed to stop the infectivity of H5N1 than other forms of influenza viruses. Even though the recommended adult dose of Tamiflu for prevention is two pills, or a total of 150 milligrams a day for 10 days, it appears this dose will not provide even marginal protection.[13]

But an apparent lack of efficacy has never deterred the pharmaceutical companies from promoting a drug or vaccine. Therefore, if it comes to pass that this research is widely accepted and higher doses are recommended during a pandemic, this will constitute an even bigger bonanza for Roche Pharmaceuticals, the Swiss company that is the sole manufacturer of Tamiflu. The numbers are overwhelming: 6.2 billion people worldwide taking two pills per day for just 10 days would require 124 *billion* pills. The average cost of a 10-day course of medicine is around $100, and if 30 times that amount is needed to make a difference...the dollars spent by countries and siphoned into Roche would be staggering.

In addition, reports that the virus is developing resistance to Tamiflu have surfaced. On February 27, 2005, a 14-year-old Vietnamese girl who had received a 75 milligram, once-a-day dose of Tamiflu for three days and then 75 milligrams twice daily for an additional seven days while hospitalized. In laboratory testing, it was determined that her isolated strain had shown resistance to the medication. (Incidentally, this patient recovered uneventfully and was discharged from the hospital on March 14, 2005.)[14]

News of a resistant strain of H5N1 caused articles to be published at lightning speed, reassuring people—and countries— that the resistant bug was merely an isolated case and that the billions of dollars being spent to stockpile the medication were not being spent in vain. Researchers noted that everyone, including

Roche, expects some resistance to Tamiflu once it is in wide use. However, if more resistance occurs, it will undoubtedly be kept under tight wraps.

Resistance has been more widely observed in children than in adults, as demonstrated by a study done in Japan in 2000 that included 50 children. When samples of influenza viruses were collected before and during treatment with Tamiflu, resistance was found in 18 percent of the viruses within four days of using the drug. Certain genes within the viruses seem to be associated with much more resistance than others. Sensitivity testing revealed that treated viruses could be 300-fold to 1,000,000-fold more resistant than viruses that had no prior exposure to Tamiflu.[15]

Resistance rates in the U.S. have not been insignificant: In pediatric trials, resistance rates were found to be 8.6 percent. This was 1.3 percent higher than those observed in the adult trials.[16] In another study in Japan, the only market to date that has embraced Tamiflu for use during seasonal influenza outbreaks, findings were consistent. That study found 16 percent of viruses developing resistance to the drug each season. "That's one in six. So I would anticipate that in H5N1-infected persons that the frequency would certainly be no less," said Dr. Frederick Hayden of the University of Virginia (also co-chair of an international network of scientists who monitor for resistance to neuraminidase inhibitors).[17]

A major concern surrounding Tamiflu-induced drug resistance is that it can lead to the potential emergence of "mutant" viruses. Mutations of the neuraminidase enzyme (N) make the virus resistant to the drug. Mutations result in the creation of a virus that is "antigenically distinct" from the original virus treated with Tamiflu. In other words, the use of Tamiflu can *cause* an antigenic drift, maybe even an antigenic shift. Once this research was published, a flurry of activity attempted to suppress or deny the implication that broad use of Tamiflu could actually *cause* the pandemic that governments and health officials are trying to avoid.

Roche resolutely denied the FDA's assertion, and pushed to smooth over the FDA's concerns that mutant viruses are "less pathogenic (less disease-causing) than wild type influenza viruses." The FDA wasn't convinced, responding, "It appears that mutant viruses may be shed at high titers [i.e., in large amounts] by some subjects before being cleared. Therefore, *this reviewer has not been reassured that these [mutant] viruses are harmless to the general population"* [Emphasis added.][18] Instead of alleviating symptoms by a meager one to two days, Tamiflu may lead to the creation of viruses that are more virulent and more aggressive than the original strain of influenza the drug is meant to inhibit.

Information about Tamiflu gets increasingly more unsettling. Evidence indicates that taking Tamiflu may increase the seriousness of the infection in people with suppressed immune systems. Tamiflu is first prescribed for the elderly and for those with chronic lung diseases based on an assumption that those persons are more likely to be seriously compromised by the flu. However, many patients with emphysema, COPD, and severe asthma are also taking drugs that suppress the immune system. There is little data to support the safety of Tamiflu in patients who are immuno-suppressed.

Further concerns about Tamiflu in kids

Additional concerns, beyond the development of aggressive mutants, have surfaced regarding Tamiflu's safety when given to children. On November 19, 2005, the FDA's Pediatric Advisory Committee met to discuss new reports of serious skin reactions, neuropsychiatric events, and deaths associated with taking Tamiflu.

According to *IMS Health*, approximately 24.4 million prescriptions for Tamiflu were dispensed between 2001 and 2005 in Japan, and 5.5 million were filled in the U.S. during that same period. Pediatric prescriptions accounted for 11.6 million in Japan versus 872,386 in the U.S.

The FDA approved Tamiflu oral capsules on October 27, 1999, for the treatment of uncomplicated acute influenza in patients over one year of age. A new indication for preventing influenza in adults and children 13 years and older was added on November 20, 2000. The liquid form of Tamiflu was approved on December 14, 2000.[19] Pediatric exclusivity was granted to Roche for Tamiflu on March 22, 2004.[20]

As part of its post-marketing surveillance efforts, the FDA

examined reports submitted to the drug Adverse Events Reporting System (AERS) database, searching for serious and non-serious adverse events that had been reported to occur in children. Because AERS is woefully underutilized by physicians, the actual number of adverse events is likely to have been much higher than actually reported. It is estimated that less than 10 percent of adverse events are reported to AERS or its vaccine equivalent, VAERS.

The query dates, from March 22, 2004, through April 22, 2005, encompassed the 13 months of use; 1,184 reports of adverse reactions were posted from sources both domestic and abroad. Nearly 16 percent of the events occurred in children (n = 190).[21]

Among the 75 pediatric reports of serious side effects, there were eight fatalities (four sudden deaths, three cardio-respiratory arrests, and one case of acute pancreatitis with cardiopulmonary arrest); 32 neuropsychiatric events; and 12 skin/hypersensitivity events. Miscellaneous other side effects were included on a list that was reviewed at the FDA meeting.[22]

Since Tamiflu's 1999 approval, an increasing number of deaths have been reported each influenza season in patients who used the drug. Of the eight children who died during the survey period, several had developed influenza, started therapy with Tamiflu, and died suddenly in their sleep.

The skin reactions reported were quite severe and included anaphylaxis, erythema multifome, and Stevens-Johnson syndrome—an extreme, potentially life-threatening immune reaction. Beyond skin reactions, the reports of neuropsychiatric events were highly disturbing and included cases of delirium, convulsions, and encephalitis. However, the most alarming adverse event was the abnormal behavior exhibited by three patients after receiving Tamiflu:

> "Two children, a 12- and a 13-year-old male, jumped out of the second floor windows of their homes after receiving two doses of Tamiflu. Head CT scans showed no abnormalities in either patient. A third case was an eight-year-old boy who also exhibited abnormal behavior when he experienced

frightening hallucinations and rushed out of his house into the street three hours after receiving his first dose of oseltamivir. He was rescued by his family from potential traffic injury."[23]

In spite of these serious reports, but true to form, the FDA voted unanimously that Tamiflu had no link to the deaths of the eight children who died. The agency chose to "continue to monitor adverse events," and that the committee would be provided with a one-year surveillance update after the flu season. This type of so-called "surveillance" is woefully inadequate. Part of the FDA's mission statement includes protecting public health by ensuring the safety of biological products, medical devices, etc. This is not ensuring safety; this is insuring the continued sale of Tamiflu. Everyone, especially parents, should be wary of using this drug. Tamiflu provides, at best, 1.5 days of relief from flu-like symptoms that will subside on their own, and it can have lethal consequences.

Rumsfeld behind the scenes

With all these problems—marginal effectiveness, serious side effects, growing viral resistance, and the possible creation of aggressive "mutant" viruses—one would think that there would be little interest in Tamiflu. But despite the apparent lack of value to the health of individuals, Roche is making colossal gains. In fact, since March 2003, LaRoche's stock rose from $78 per share to a whopping $208 per share by the end of 2005. But behind the obvious profits to the manufacturer, an intriguing paper trail has been uncovered that leads directly to the U.S. government. It appears that one government official, in particular, is poised to gain personally from the billion dollar purchases of Tamiflu.

Tamiflu was developed and patented in 1996 by the California biotech firm Gilead Sciences. The world marketing rights to manufacture the drug were then signed over to Hoffmann-LaRoche (located in Switzerland), in exchange for a 10 percent royalty on every dose sold. That's not such big news, but the fact that Donald

Rumsfeld was the chairman of the board of Gilead Sciences during the time that Tamiflu was developed is huge news. He held that position from 1997 until early 2001, when he resigned to join the current administration as secretary of defense.

When Rumsfeld left Gilead's board, the company's stock price was around $7 per share. Since March 2003, Gilead's stock soared, in part, due to the purchase of $58 million worth of Tamiflu by global governments in July of that year. The increase translates into tens of millions for Rumsfeld—a hefty 720 percent windfall of profit. *Morningstar, Inc.* reported that when bird flu rose in prominence during the summer of 2005, Rumsfeld considered selling all of his Gilead stock, but on the advice of a private securities lawyer who refused to be identified, Rumsfeld was advised to keep the stock and make known to the public his "recusal" from avian flu decisions "in order to avoid being accused of a sale based on insider information."[24]

That's such great spin it sounds like it came from a top New York PR firm. It is curious that the secretary waited until October 26, 2005, before issuing this official press statement, especially since this wasn't the first time that Rumsfeld has been on the inside track and made millions from drug company deals with the government.

Tracking the past

In 1976, while serving as the secretary of defense to President Ford, Rumsfeld clearly contributed to Ford's quick decision to produce and distribute the ill-fated swine flu vaccine. What possible benefits the secretary obtained through participation is unknown, as political records of his tenure with the Ford administration are unavailable to the general public.

The current administration has another member with experience in pandemic planning. During the Ford administration, Richard Cheney held the position of deputy chief of staff and was then promoted to chief of staff when Rumsfeld became secretary of defense in November 1975. (As a point of history, this was the same time that George Bush, Sr. was appointed head of the CIA.) The Ford Library collection admits that, although senior staff members met on a daily basis, the large number of meetings that Cheney attended is barely documented, with only a few scattered notes appearing in the files.[25]

In addition, the files from Rumsfeld's term with Ford are not available. A strong argument can be made that both Rumsfeld and Cheney were present and contributed to the push for swine flu mass vaccination. In all likelihood they are doing the same thing now regarding the bird flu.

Upon Ford's defeat, and the arrival of Jimmy Carter and the Democrats to the White House, Rumsfeld returned to the private sector to become president and then later chairman of the board for G.D. Searle & Co., a worldwide pharmaceutical company.

Rumsfeld's life, prior to his arrival at Searle, has been called a great Midwestern success story. Born in Chicago, he was a wrestling champ at New Trier High School (class of 1950) and at Princeton (1954), a navy pilot, and a congressman. Throughout his career, Rumsfeld has been known as a highly ambitious, tough operator with a reputation for ferociously pursuing what he wanted.[26] Although he had next to no experience in private business, what he brought to the table for Searle was government ties and an insider's grasp of the workings in Washington. All of these attributes were exactly what Searle needed.

Since 1965, the company had been attempting to bring its artificial sweetener, aspartame, to market. Aspartame was originally developed as a drug for gastric ulcers, but then the research scientist who was working with the compound inadvertently tasted it and found it to be extraordinarily sweet. On further testing, the sweetness was found to be 180 times greater than the taste of sugar. Searle immediately shifted the focus from developing a limited-use pharmaceutical product for ulcers to a "calorie-free" additive that could be used in thousands of products and purchased by billions of repeat customers worldwide.

However, despite Searle's spending of millions on research and drug applications, the FDA refused to approve aspartame for use. From the beginning, the approval process had been fraught with problems ranging from rejections due to inconsistent safety studies to grand jury probes investigating fabricated data.

Consumer groups had filed legal proceedings to stop its use due to serious concerns. Studies had demonstrated that aspartame caused brain cancers in experimental animals. There didn't seem to be much hope for getting this potential blockbuster approved.

The outlook improved, however, with the return of the Republican Party to the White House. When Ronald Reagan took the oath of office as the fortieth president on January 21, 1981, Rumsfeld was poised to move the approval of aspartame through to completion. He was so confident in his party connections that, according to former G.D. Searle salesperson, Patty Wood-Allott, he told his sales force "he would call in all his markers" and "no matter what," he would see to it that aspartame would be approved during that year.[27] Politics would supersede safety as reports from aspartame research showed disastrous consequences on the health of a large number of experimental animals.

Moving aspartame to approval

Four days after Reagan's inauguration, previous FDA commissioner, Jere E. Goyan, was replaced by professor and Defense Department contract researcher, Dr. Arthur Hayes. No clear reason can be found in the public record why he was selected over other candidates, but it was rumored he was "hand-picked" due to his close ties with Rumsfeld during his previous tenure as secretary of defense.

Despite all information to the contrary regarding aspartame's supposed "safety," Hayes overruled the Public Board of Inquiry, disregarded scientific warnings, ignored several laws in the Food Drug and Cosmetic Act, and in July 1981 approved aspartame for use in dry foods. Just as Rumsfeld had predicted, the approval had been completed within the year. In 1983, the chemical was approved for use in consumer soft drinks. Today, aspartame is found in more than 5,000 products under the brand names Equal® and NutraSweet®.[28]

Attorney and consumer advocate James Turner, who fought the aspartame approval process for years, commented that for Hayes to arrive so quickly to the conclusion that aspartame was safe, he had "firewalked a path through a mass of scientific mismanagement, improper procedures, wrong conclusions, and general scientific inexactness," meaning he had been given marching orders which he carried perfectly to completion, turning a blind-eye to both science and the law.

Shortly after the additive was approved, Commissioner Hayes was forced to leave the FDA after being investigated for accepting a bribe from General Foods, a major user of aspartame. Criminal investigations aside, Hayes soon became dean of New York Medical College and was hired by Burson-Marsteller, Searle's public relations firm (which also represented several of NutraSweet's major users) as senior scientific consultant and medical advisor.[29]

The rewards for those involved with the approval of aspartame were huge. In 1985, Searle was purchased by Monsanto, and lawyer Robert Shapiro, who navigated the name change from aspartame to NutraSweet®, was named president of Monsanto. After the sale was finalized, Rumsfeld reportedly received a $12 million bonus.[30]

> For more in-depth information on this topic, see *Excitotoxins: The Taste That Kills*, by Russell Baylock, MD, and *Deadly Deception: The Story of Aspartame*, by Mary Nash Stoddard

The complete story of aspartame is far beyond the scope of this text, but a few points deserve to be highlighted. In 1992, FDA Commissioner Dr. David Kessler approved its use in heated food, such as baked goods, despite research that shows heated aspartame is converted to formaldehyde. Four years later it was approved for use in all foods. After completing the approval process, Kessler resigned from the FDA to take a position as dean of the Yale School of Medicine. This is another example of how deeply politics, big business, and medical education are connected.

Rumsfeld's Next Big Prize

Gilead Science was founded in June 1987 by Michael Riordan to develop products for the treatment of viral diseases including human immunodeficiency virus (HIV), hepatitis B virus, herpes simplex virus, and human papillomavirus (HPV). Its first FDA-approved product, Vistide® (cidofovir), was an injectable medicine approved in 1996 for the treatment of eye infections caused by cytomegalovirus (CMV) in patients with AIDS.

Even before 9/11, many companies had been working to find drugs that would be useful to protect against acts of bioterrorism, particularly smallpox. More than 700 compounds were tested for activity against the virus; of these, at least 20 were found to hold promise against vaccinia and variola viruses in vitro (in a test tube). Vistide was among this group. Early in 2001, a license for using Vistide as an investigational new drug for the treatment of an acute smallpox infection and the management of side effects associated with smallpox (vaccinia) vaccinations was filed with the FDA. This was another boon for Rumsfeld, as he had been chairman of the board for Gilead Sciences from 1993 to 2000.

But Gilead's revenue from Vistide was small potatoes compared to the lottery-level winnings that came through the U.S. government's recommendation to purchase Tamiflu. On October 6, 2005, the Pentagon announced it would begin stockpiling large quantities of Tamiflu for members of the military. As secretary of defense, Rumsfeld was perfectly positioned to play a role in this decision despite his pronouncement that he had recused himself.

Interestingly, two days later *The Boston Globe* reported that Roche announced its plans to build a plant in the U.S. to make Tamiflu, saying and would consider licensing its manufacture to other companies "in the face of a possible flu pandemic."[32] The FDA had approved an additional capsule manufacturing site in the U.S., adding to its network of more than a dozen plants worldwide. In addition, CEO of Roche Pharma Division William M. Burns said that the company was prepared to discuss all available options, including granting sub-licenses, with any government or private company who approach us to manufacture Tamiflu or collaborate with us in its manufacturing.

No doubt, this was music to Rumsfeld's ears. He will continue to benefit as the plans for Tamiflu expand and profits compound with each pill sold.

The most dangerous untruths are truths
moderately distorted.
~Georg Christoph Lichtenberg, Physicist

Chapter 12: How the Current Hype Began

Starting points:
- A petting zoo, a small boy, and the CDC

Stockpiling drugs, the specter of mandatory vaccination, WHO mandates. How did this all begin?

The bird flu hype appeared on the world stage in May 1997 through an ironically innocent setting. A Hong Kong pre-school had set up a small petting zoo on its grounds, making a home for five chickens and eight ducks. The children were, of course, delighted to spend time with their new feathered friends. Several days after the mini school aviary began, a three-year-old boy in the class began to cough. The illness and fever progressed rapidly, and the boy's parents rushed him to Victoria Hospital where he was admitted with pneumonia and respiratory distress.

Six days later the child died suddenly from complications that included Reye's syndrome, adult respiratory distress syndrome, and multiple organ system failure. During the boy's hospital stay, attending physicians noted that he had been treated with aspirin. The doctors requested an autopsy to determine why the boy had died, but the results were perplexing. Pathologists found no underlying immunodeficiency or cardiopulmonary disease that would have contributed to the boy's death. Even more confounding was that a virus isolated from a tracheal aspirate could not be identified.

It wasn't until three months later (August, 1997) that the virus was confirmed by a reference laboratory in the Netherlands and by the CDC in the United States to be avian influenza A virus, H5N1, subsequently named A/Hong Kong/156/97. In a report published later, researchers held that this particular bird flu virus had not previously caused infection in humans.[1]

Teams from the WHO and the CDC descended on Hong Kong to determine how the boy had been exposed to the virus and to assess the subsequent potential public health impact. According to investigators, one of the chickens in the petting zoo had died several days before the child's symptoms had appeared. It was postulated that the exposure to the ill bird or its feces provided a means for the virus to "jump species" and infect the boy.

Is this sounding familiar?

In the following days, there was no shortage of tension as officials scrambled to determine if the virus had been contracted by others who had been exposed to the ill child. Sweeping investigations of the birds in the surrounding area revealed that three outbreaks of H5N1 had occurred in poultry farms in the Hong Kong New Territory earlier in 1997. Approximately 2,000 human samples were collected from people who had been in contact with the boy, the animals in the school's petting zoo, and the birds from the rural areas.

Significantly, none of the dead child's four closest relatives tested positive for antibodies that would indicate the presence of the H5N1 virus. However, a few others who had been in contact with the child had positive tests. Nearly 2 percent of healthcare workers who cared for him, 1 percent of his classmates, and 2 percent of the family's neighbors showed evidence of having contact with the "new virus." Despite the presence of H5N1 antibodies in their blood, *all of these people were symptom-free.*[2]

A second case of H5N1 infection was confirmed in Hong Kong on November 26, 1997, and more cases appeared throughout December. The samples taken from birds during this outbreak were identical matches to the viruses collected from the deceased child. There were a total of 18 confirmed cases affecting eight males and 10 females, ranging in age from one to 60, with half of those afflicted below the age of 12.

The news of the direct bird-to-human transmission sent a chill throughout the medical and scientific community: This was reported to be the first documented isolation of H5N1 in humans. This was all public health officials around the globe needed to hear. Even though there was no evidence of human-to-human transmission and no further human infections were found, they believed the potential for the next pandemic had arrived.

Continued outbreaks

A few sporadic outbreaks of highly pathogenic avian influenza continued throughout the world between 1997 and late 2002. However, beginning late in 2003 and throughout early 2004, outbreaks of H5N1 were reported among poultry concentrated in a few countries, mostly in Southeast Asia: Cambodia, Indonesia, Laos, Thailand, and Vietnam. Approximately 45 people tested positive for the H5N1 virus and a handful died. The finger-pointing began as to the cause of the problem, and family farmers throughout the region were placed directly in the crosshairs.

A poor man's field may produce abundant food,
but injustice sweeps it away.
~Proverbs 13:23

Chapter 13: The Killing Fields

Starting points:
- The recommended method for containing outbreaks— Kill all the birds
- The plan to eliminate the family farm
- Tyson in Thailand: The model for global agribusiness

I t bears repeating that despite all the recent media attention, avian influenza—even H5N1 infection—is not new. WHO records show 21 reported outbreaks worldwide of highly pathogenic avian influenza since 1959. The majority struck in Europe with a few occurring in Mexico and Canada. Of the total, five resulted in significant spread to poultry farms and resulted in severe economic losses to regional economies due to the slaughter of millions of chickens.[1]

In most Southeast Asian countries, raising poultry as a backyard operation has been a common practice for centuries. In fact, 80 percent of the world's poultry, including at least 60 percent of China's estimated 13.2 billion chickens, are raised in free-range style. The activity is both a means for supplementing income and providing food for the family.[2] Rarely would one find village fowl being kept under the intensive, caged system the way U.S. birds are raised.

Village chickens form an integral part of village life and have an important social value in some countries. As the term "scavenging village chickens" describes, many birds obtain their feed from their surrounding environment, food composed mainly of fallen grains, worms, insects, and table and kitchen scraps, as well as local weeds and grasses. Chickens of all ages are usually fed twice a day, early in the morning before the birds are released and in the evening when they come back to roost. Breeding stock is locally raised and contains local genetics; males and females mate naturally and randomly since birds of all ages and both sexes roam freely. Flock sizes vary, but on average families raise 20 to 50 birds between the ages of one day to about three years.[3]

Killing the flocks to bring influenza outbreaks under control remains the first course of action recommended by the Food and Agriculture Organization of the United Nations (FAO), the World Organization for Animal Health (OIE), and the WHO. These organizations advocate the killing of all birds that have been exposed to avian influenza virus subtypes H5 and H7, even if the chickens show no signs of illness. Culling is based on the 1920s assumption that once a viral outbreak has occurred among a flock, the only way to eliminate the virus is to eliminate the host.[4]

While international bodies call for the massacre of all birds exposed to highly pathogenic influenza viruses, there are no international regulations governing how the birds are to be killed. Methods include burning, drowning, gassing, and live burial. Throughout the world tens of millions of birds have been brutally killed. In Bali 228,000 chickens were reportedly either burned alive or kicked and beaten to death. In Thailand more than ten million birds were destroyed, most by burying them alive. "As soon as the first 500 died, we had to bury the other 20,000 alive," a Thai farmer told a reporter.[5]

The most commonly used killing method has been stuffing live birds into plastic bags, where they suffocate as they are buried alive in mass graves. On smaller farms, chickens have had their necks wrung or have been bashed to death with a stick prior to being buried. Workers have reported being traumatized by killing so many struggling chickens, particularly over the emotional protests of local farmers.[6] In Turkey, slaughter has drawn strong protests from locals, many of whom surrendered their animals only after officials warned that those who hid their fowl would face a prison term of up to six months and a hefty fine.[7]

Descending on small farms and in front of tearful owners, hundreds of soldiers and state agricultural workers walk along the rows of cages, pulling out the struggling, squawking birds, stuffing them into sacks. "I pray for

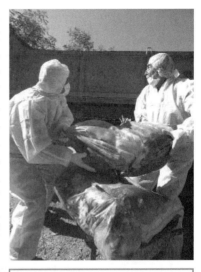

Members of a verterinary team load a truck with bags of culled poultry in southern Macedonia's village of Mogila. October 2005. (AP Photo by Boris Grdanoski)

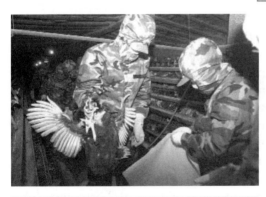

Chinese soldiers from the People's Armed Police Force slaughter chickens in notheast China's Liaoning Povince. November 2005. (AP Photo by Xinhua, Xie Huanchi)

the chickens every night. But when I wake up the next morning, I have to do the same job again. It's no different from being an executioner," one of the state workers told a reporter.[8]

The close living conditions of farmers with their poultry are being blamed for evolution of the highly pathogenic strains. The theory is that side-by-side domestication between people and poultry increases the contact time between humans and fowl, increasing the odds that an aggressive form of the virus will emerge, "jump species," and start the next worldwide pandemic. However, something just doesn't add up. The vast majority of the chickens and ducks that have been brutally murdered have been healthy—showing no signs of illness. Neither have their owners shown any sign of being sick. Is there another reason for culling more than 200 million birds in poor countries? Who has the most to gain by the elimination of the independent family farm?

Agribusiness plan: The end of the family-run farm?

Prior to 1930, U.S. poultry production was confined primarily to small, rural farms. Not unlike the situation in Southeast Asia, China, and Eastern Europe, free-range chickens were raised for their eggs and occasionally slaughtered for their meat. But by mid-century, large corporate entities had begun to edge out the family farmer. While there were still 2,500 independent egg-producing companies in the U.S. in 1987, by February 2004, the number had been reduced to a mere 260. Currently, almost 95 percent of all farms in the U.S. are controlled by agribusiness.[9]

Similarly, there has been a move toward the semi-intensive farming system throughout the far eastern regions of the world where birds are kept in tightly enclosed areas for shelter and feeding. A study by Ramlah and Shukor (1987) showed that rural farmers in Malaysia mainly practiced the free-range system, followed by the semi-intensive system (15.4 percent) and the intensive cage system (1 percent). And as industrialized farming has become more popular among throughout Malaysia in recent years, a few are rearing as many as 10,000 birds per farm.

The industrial integration of the family farm began in 1957 by two Harvard Business School economists—Ray Goldberg and John Davis—who envisioned a concentrated, vertically integrated food business that streamlined food production from the farm to the grocers' shelves. A system designed first for American farms and then to be applied to the rest of the world, the new concept was named "agribusiness"—defined as "the sum total of all operations involved in the manufacture and distribution of farm supplies, production operations on the farm, and the storage, processing, and distribution of farm commodities and the items made from them."[10] This definition, establishing agriculture as an industry, would go far beyond simply growing crops and raising animals. The goal was to create an assembly line for food production, creating maximum profits for the agribusiness conglomerates that would come to own or control every aspect of the farm.

Throughout the industrial and technological age, capitalism and science have blended with stunning ease and speed, but the results haven't always been pretty. In the U.S., the mega-purveyors of poultry in agribusiness, Cargill, Perdue Farms, ConAgra Poultry, GoldKist Inc., and Tyson Foods, control the vast majority of the poultry industry in the world. Leaving little doubt that profitability is among their most important directives, researchers have severely commoditized the poultry industry through genetic interventions that are unsettling. Genetically altered chickens and turkeys grow twice as fast and twice as large as their non-genetically modified counterparts and are referred to as "units" and "machines."

Even though the modern chicken industry claims it is focused on safety and food quality, even a cursory examination of the business suggests otherwise. The animals are nothing more than products and a means to make money. Since 1990, when for the first time ever in the U.S. people consumed more chicken than beef, the broiler chicken and egg sectors of the poultry industry have recorded the fastest growth rates in their histories. And the trends continue to move upward. Exports of eggs and egg products rose to 103.2 million dozen during the first half of 2005, compared with 61.6 million dozen during the same period in 2004. To keep up with the demand, hens that once lived freely and laid eggs occasionally have been bred to produce under exploitive, artificial conditions. Through a combination of genetic and chemical manipulation, hens are capable of producing an abnormally large number of eggs—250 per year— in contrast to the normal one or two clutches of 10 to 12 eggs annually.[12]

It is astonishing to discover that there are no federal laws to regulate the raising, transporting, and slaughtering of poultry in the

U.S. The industry opposes legislation that would allow for the humane sacrifice of poultry, claiming that hens cannot be "economically rendered insensible to pain" prior to having their throats cut or being decapitated. Since there is little reason to assume the industry will make the reforms without good cause, conditions will remain dire for the birds and workers alike.[13]

In addition to the repugnant treatment of animals, employees who work in slaughterhouses owned by the agri-giants also fare poorly. Poultry processing is one of the two most dangerous industries in the U.S., according to a U.S. Government Accountability Office (GAO) report from January 7, 2005. (The other is the meat packing industry.) Poultry workers endure hazardous conditions involving loud noise, sharp tools, and dangerous machinery. The job entails standing for long periods, wielding knives and hooks toward carcasses moving along production lines at the dizzying rate of 91 chickens per minute, the maximum allowable speed. This frantic, repetitive work leads to one of the highest rates of injury and illness of any industry. As expected, common injuries include cuts, cumulative trauma, and injuries sustained from falls, but more serious injuries have occurred including fractures and amputations.[14]

Currently, the U.S. is the world's largest producer and exporter of poultry meat—chicken, turkey, and duck—with production valued at nearly $23 billion annually. Of the companies that dominate the world markets, Tyson Foods is by far the largest, both nationally and internationally. Tyson processes 25 percent more than its closest rival, Pilgrim's Pride, and almost three times the volume of the next closest rival, GoldKist.[15]

The Top 10 Poultry Producers in the U.S.

1. Tyson Foods
2. Pilgrim's Pride Corporation
3. GoldKist
4. Perdue Farms
5. Sanderson Farms
6. Wayne Farms
7. Mountaine Farms
8. Foster Farms
9. OK Foods, Inc.
10. Peco Foods

U.S. Poultry & Egg Association (February 2005)

Forbes Magazine once described Tyson Foods as one of those "undeniably formidable business juggernauts, whose mind-boggling concentrations of wealth and influence have everything to do with a no-holds-barred, unfettered approach to free enterprise."[16] Headquartered in Springdale, Arkansas, Tyson operates 300 facilities in 26 states and employs more than 120,000 people. With offices in 22 nations, Tyson exported to more than 80 foreign countries in fiscal 2002. Major export markets included Canada, Mexico, European Union, Russia, Japan, China, and South Korea.[17]

Accused of creating agreements with farmers that border on near-indentured servitude, Tyson supplies the farmer with the baby chicks and everything necessary to raise them, including feed, vaccines, and medications. Even the necessary technology and technical services are included–all in a massive attempt to streamline production. In this industrialized chicken arrangement referred to as "factory farming," the farmer assumes all the risks of day-to-day operations, and if the birds get sick or die he is responsible for the costs.[18] But however egregious this arrangement appears to be for farmers, the industry giant has benefited to such a great extent it is looking for people and birds to exploit in other parts of the world. To that end, it appears that the small farmers in the rest of the world may be the next target to become low wage workers for Tyson and similar mega-corporations.

Tyson in Thailand

In the span of just a few years, the Thai poultry industry has grown from nothing more than a patchwork of backyard chicken producers to an advanced production system, thanks to its adaptation of the Tyson model. By 2003 Thailand had become the fourth-largest poultry exporter in the world.

Up to 90 percent of Thai chicken production is exported mainly to the European Union and Japan through the poultry powerhouse in Southeast Asia, the Bangkok-based Charoen Pokphand (CP). A multinational conglomerate employing more than 100,000 people in 20 countries, CP maintains food production as its core business, but its activities range from seeds and telecoms to the franchise of 7/Eleven retail stores. The CP Group has the ambition to become "the kitchen of the world," a mission commandeered by the government on behalf of the entire country.[19] The exponential growth has the full support of Thailand's Prime Minister, Thaksin Shinawatram, reportedly one of the richest businessmen in the country.

With this much political and economic clout behind the multinational corporation, much was at risk with the appearance of H5N1 in Thailand's fowl in 2004. In an attempt to suppress information that the virus had been found in local flocks, high government officials reassured the prime minister that Thailand was definitely free of outbreaks. A campaign of massive proportions to protect one of the country's primary industries consisted of so many cover-ups, incompetencies, and outright lies. As reported in *The Bangkok Post* on February 6, 2004:

> "'Before November, we were processing about 90,000 chickens a day. But from November to January, we had to kill about 130,000 daily.' Workers were asked to work overtime to hurry the processing, stating, 'We saw many diseased chickens arriving and were ordered to process them, even if they had already died from the illness. It's our job to cut the birds up,' said one employee. 'It was obvious they were ill: their organs were swollen. We didn't know what the disease was, but we understood that management

was rushing to process the chicken before getting any
veterinary inspection. We stopped eating [chicken]
in October.'"[20]

After two months of denials, the government was finally forced
to admit the presence of the H5N1 virus on January 23, 2004, and
confessed that two people had tested positive for bird flu, with
another three under observation. Local papers soon began reporting
that a few people suspected of having the disease had died, and the
Agriculture Ministry was forced to publicly admit that more than six
million chickens had already been culled. Local newspapers
exposed officials who had been aware of the presence of Highly
Pathogenic Avian Influenza (HPAI) since November 2003, but were
told to "keep it quiet and blame the culling of poultry on an outbreak
of chicken cholera and bronchitis."[21]

Protection of the mega-poultry producers became blatant when,
in spite of the presence of infected poultry, Prime Minister Thaksin
engaged in a personal crusade to encourage people to eat their
favorite chicken dishes. Massive public relations campaigns were
instituted to convince Thai citizens that eating chicken was a "patriotic
duty." The campaign included a personal plea from the governor of
Bangkok, who said, "If Thais don't eat Thai chicken, how can we
expect others to buy our chicken?"[22]

At the same time as officials were scrambling to find ever more
novel ways to encourage chicken consumption, Thai troops and
about 60 prisoners from local jails, donning rubber gloves, shower
caps, and safety masks, were dispatched to 41 of the country's 76
rural provinces to kill and bury poultry belonging to local
farmers. When the H5N1 virus was detected, a "red zone" was
declared around the farm. All the poultry in the zone and within a
certain radius of the zone were killed, ostensibly to prevent the
spread of the virus. However, some farmers reported dead chickens
had been found on farms where no red zone had been declared,
lending support to the suspicion that authorities were protecting
some farmers over others.[23] The accusations seemed to be
substantiated when CP-owned farmers were promised full

compensation and rapid replacement of stock, and local farmers were left to wonder if government-promised compensation would ever come.

Authorities estimate more than 40,000 small and medium-sized open-air poultry farms are scattered throughout Thailand, and most have been raided by chicken marauders. Independent farmers were not as fortunate as CP farmers; they received under-market compensation by local authorities if they received anything at all.[24] To gain their cooperation, the prime minister had promised to "turn the crisis into opportunity." But helping the local farmer reestablish his business wasn't exactly the opportunity that the Thai government seemed to have in mind.

Chia Ek Chow from mainland China (who adopted a Thai name, Dhanin Chearavanont), brought Tyson-style farming to Thailand in 1971 through a partnership with Arbor Acres, a subsidiary of Aviagen Group, the company that controls one-third of the genetic stock of all the broiler chickens in the world. Replacement stock for local farmers no doubt came from either Aviagen or Tyson's Cobb-Vantress; both breeds have been genetically manipulated.

Throughout the crisis, the chairman of the CP Group, Dhanin Chearavanont, continued to push his agenda that closed farms, where chickens have minimal contact with humans and no contact with wild birds, were "bird flu free" zones. His insistence that industrial farming was the "safest way to produce chickens" was embraced unconditionally by the Thai government, even though his claims were more than unfounded—they were actually outright lies. During the same time that the government was going public with its admissions and assurances (February 2004), the army had been mobilized to kill 117,000 birds on a CP-owned industrial chicken farm, one of the largest in the province.[25]

Eliminating the independent farms, one by one

Proving that burdensome bureaucracies are not unique to western culture, the Thai government launched a plan to "modernize national poultry farming." This included setting new standards and stiff regulations for independent farmers, part of which would require them to register every chicken. Mandatory upgrades included building industrial-grade poultry houses, an incinerator for dead birds, and special coops for sick ones. These hefty new standards were required before farmers could receive replacement stock for their culled birds. When farmers lamented that they could not afford to abide by the new rules, three state banks stepped forward offering loans for the farm upgrades. Because of the steep investments required to build industrial farms (up to 10 million baht per farm, or $252,750 in U.S. currency) most small, independent raisers were wiped out. Reportedly, more than 1,000 farmers throughout Thailand gave up their farm business due to the financial hardship imposed by the new regulations.[26]

ANIMAL REGISTRATION TO START IN THE U.S.

In March, 2006, The National Animal Identification System, which has been under development by the U.S. Department of Agriculture since 2002—with help from an agribusiness giants Cargill and Monsanto—was announced in the U.S. Under this system, animal owners and livestock handlers will be required to attach microchips or other ID tags to their animals and birds. They will be monitored throughout their lifetimes by a centralized computer network. The system has three phases. First, farmers and producers will be required to register the barns, factories, slaughterhouses, and even homes where their animals reside and/or are processed. Second, those animals will be assigned a 15-digit federal ID number and a tag that, in some cases, would be implanted into the animal as a radio-frequency identification (RFID) device. Third, data on each animal's whereabouts would be compiled and regularly updated through a centralized computer network, which the USDA expects to be implemented on a national scale by 2009. The USDA has allocated more than $60 million to help states with animal-ID programs.

One of the first steps in creating indentured servants—whether it is personal indebtedness to multinationals or a country's obligations to the World Bank—is to force them into debt. Forcing farmers to borrow money to comply with regulations designed to benefit agribusiness and CP should leave little doubt about the intent.

As farmers watched, their livelihoods literally vanished in a matter of hours at the behest of the government's sweeping mandates. "It's all very well for the government to talk about 40 baht (US$1) per chicken in compensation, but that is only enough to live on, to get food to eat. Our whole farms have disappeared and now we have nothing left. Will they pay for us to restock? We need to wait and see what the government has to offer, but I haven't seen any money yet," a local farmer told reporters. "In this district there are only a few families who have received compensation, but nearly everyone has lost their chickens. We have big loans to pay."[27]

For many, chicken farming has been their only means of earning a living, and the social impact of such an aggressive move toward industrial farming will take a serious toll on the already over-burdened economic system. In spite of the extreme success of the national chicken business, few local Thai farmers have benefited. In fact, while the value of food exports increased by 52 percent between 1995 and 2000, the average debt per farming household increased by 51 percent. Even a top CP executive candidly admitted that the number of independent farmers was "likely to decrease" as a result of the new standards implemented in the wake of the bird flu outbreak, making the inequities even greater.[28]

The conversion of farmers to corporate agribusiness workers has moved at a rapid rate throughout Thailand. As of mid-2004, the Tyson-styled CP Group had nearly 10,000 contracted poultry farms in operation, and that number will likely escalate. Corporate farming will continue to capitalize on the H5N1 outbreaks as a way to eliminate the independent farm. An organic farmer explained how farmers become dependent on CP:

> "The company comes and makes wonderful promises to the farmers. In my village, they convinced many of us to start raising chicken for them. Then the exploitation comes. Farmers have to invest a lot of money at the beginning. There is a guaranteed price, but CP always finds a way to pay less, arguing that

the farmers didn't respect the standards, that the quality is not good, that the production is late. Contract farmers become very indebted; they sometimes have a 300,000 baht debt (US$7,500). Personally, I will never enter into a contract with CP. They destroy small farmers with false promises."[29]

Ms. Kulnipa Panton, president of the trade union at a chicken processing factory in Rangsit/Bangkok, said that workers are trying to establish a union because the current slaughterhouse and farming policies are structured against the poor. Many groups across the country are convinced that the bird flu outbreak is being used to push forward a vertically integrated farming agenda, instead of using the crisis as an opportunity to develop production systems that would benefit local farmers, workers, and consumers.[30]

Tyson Foods, CP, and other food giants are positioned to capitalize on the opportunity presented by bird flu, installing industrial chicken farming throughout the region. A whole new group of potential "serfs" are available throughout these countries, and the mega-businesses are in a position to make that happen.

Agribusiness in Vietnam

Of all the countries in Southeast Asia, Vietnam has had the most outbreaks of H5N1. In February 2005, the country's largest city, Ho Chi Minh City (formerly Saigon), killed 100 percent of the poultry there. "Once the outbreak has receded, we will allow farms to hatch eggs again, but poultry farming will be tightly controlled," said Bui Quang Anh, director of the Agriculture Ministry's Animal Health Department. Located near the Mekong Delta, South Vietnam's former capital has had repeated outbreaks of bird flu since December 2003.[31]

The slaughter of all chickens and ducks continued throughout 2005 in an attempt to meet deadlines imposed by the government to kill all the poultry inside major cities. No bird escaped being killed, including pet starlings and parrots. Hanoi poultry farmers were compensated 15,000 dong (US$0.95) for each destroyed duck, which cost 40,000 dong (US$2.53) to raise. "It is our entire fortune plus bank loans," said 43-year-old Nguyen Van Tan, who owned 3,500 ducks and has raised poultry since 1990. "We want the compensation early to change jobs, to restore my life, and for my children's meals and study."[32]

At a WHO preparedness meeting in Geneva held November 7–9, 2005, the heads of countries around the world pledged resources to pandemic prevention. The vice-minister of agriculture and rural development from Vietnam, Dr. Bui Ba Bong, committed to huge changes, including the complete restructuring of the local poultry industry and the industrialization of the poultry sector. Bans on raising poultry in urban areas were developed, as were bans on the commingling of free-ranging waterfowl and farm fowl. In exchange for revamping the production, slaughter, sale, and consumption of poultry, i.e., for creating industrial poultry farms, he requested US$50million for 2005–6. An additional sum of US$100million was requested for continued surveillance activities through 2010. (Note: Exchange rate in 2005 was US$1 equals $15,000 VND.)[33]

In Vietnam, where the bulk of poultry is still raised by backyard producers, the impact of the mass culling of family revenue and food will only partly be offset by government compensation. Survey data show that in Vietnam the poorest quintile of households relies more than three times as much on poultry income as does the richest quintile. Changing the way poultry is raised will create the same hardships for the local Vietnamese as it has for rural Thai farmers, and the outcomes will no doubt be the same.[34]

Agribusiness takeovers: Not a "coincidence"

Mergers and acquisitions between agribusiness and pharmaceutical companies occur at a dizzying pace, and the scope of involvement is massive. As the new joint ventures come and go, keeping it all straight and current is nearly impossible. Horizontal and vertical integration, connecting food production with food processing for retail sales, is complex. The diagram seen on page 159, created in 1999 by Mary Hendrickson, PhD, assistant professor and director of the food

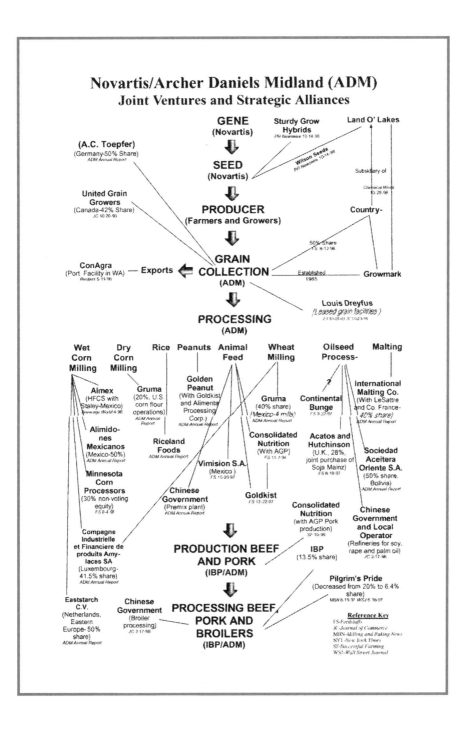

Novartis/Archer Daniels Midland (ADM)
Joint Ventures and Strategic Alliances

159

Circles Networking Project at the University of Missouri, gives an appreciation for the complexity of the food processing industry. For example, the agrochemical divisions of Novartis and AstraZeneca merged forming Syngenta, the world's largest research organization for genetically modified seeds. Another company, IBP Corporation, no longer exists; it is now wholly owned by Tyson Foods.

Engineering takeovers of companies to expand its global market share, Tyson Foods has been in the limelight more than once for its many corporate maneuvers. To call the company opportunistic may be a distinct understatement. For example, *USA Today* reported that during the summer of 2001 Tyson had the most to gain from the widespread outbreaks of foot-and-mouth disease among cattle in the U.K. Caused by at least seven separate viruses and many viral subtypes, foot-and-mouth disease wreaked havoc across the world, even though it is a non-fatal disease and there were no reported cases in humans. Symptoms in animals included fever; vesicles on the nose and mouth; thick saliva; painful tongue; and lameness or reluctance to move due to sores on the hooves. Some commentators described the effects as "little more than a common cold" in animals.

Daily reports of foot-and-mouth disease outbreaks resulted in the culling of more than six million animals in the U.K alone. The economic aftermath for the government was £3 billion (US$5.2 billion), and the impact on tourism and the rural economy climbed to more than £5billion (US$8.7 billion). The government's policy was called "contiguous culling," meaning that all animals within a 1.86 miles radius (3-kilometer radius) of an "infected premise" were ordered to be killed, whether diseased or not.[35]

Similar to the killing that has been ordered to eliminate poultry, raids on U.K. farms occurred throughout 2001 to eliminate cattle, sheep, and other hoofed animals. Juanita Wilson owns an animal sanctuary in southern Scotland. Her story was reported on April 22, 2002, by *World Net Daily:*

> "'The raid on my premises started minutes before 6 o'clock in the morning [on May 11]. There were at least 30 policemen—we've never been able to ascertain how many exactly, but there were two mini-buses full

and a lot of individual cars, plus the slaughter team. They had come to kill my animals and were blocking the roads to keep the media and protesters from getting to me. It's something I'll never forget.' The animals were hauled away by slaughter teams driving white trucks, dubbed 'cull wagons.' Traversing the countryside, the wagons carted away tens of thousands of animals that were buried in mass pits and destroyed by funeral pyres."[36]

The elimination of massive numbers of U.K. cattle positioned Tyson perfectly to pounce on its long-sought acquisition, IBP Corporation, having tried unsuccessfully four times to purchase it. The international slaughter of cattle during the foot-and-mouth outbreak reduced IBP profits to the distinct benefit of Tyson. In 2001 Tyson Foods, America's largest poultry producer, acquired IBP, the U.K.'s largest beef processor, in a hostile takeover that included $4.7 billion in cash, stock, and debt. [37]

Alarms were immediately voiced by president of the U.S. National Farmers Organization, Paul Olson. Speaking for other growers and ranchers, he voiced concern that the Tyson-IBP merger would represent an "unprecedented agricultural concentration" of power. Fears were stated that the merger gave Tyson so much monopolistic control in the international markets over poultry, beef, and pork that independent producers would be completely driven out of business.

The ranchers' outrage was also shared by Senator Paul Wellstone (D-MN), who stated, "This merger would create a company with control over 30 percent of the beef market, 33 percent of the chicken market, and 18 percent of the pork market." Before his untimely death, Wellstone pledged to push the Bush administration's Department of Justice to scrutinize the merger; since his death, no investigation has ever been launched.[38]

Another example of Tyson's business practices, the takeover of another competitor, Hudson Foods, was succinctly described by Steven Ransom in his on-line article, "Without Bars:"[39]

"In 1997, Tyson Foods expressed interest in buying beef giant Hudson Foods. Hudson declined the Tyson offer. Very soon after the rejection of Tyson's bid, a government inspectorate task force under the control of Agriculture Secretary Dan Glickman 'visited' Hudson Foods, where they very conveniently 'found' evidence of *E.coli* bacteria contamination. By the time Glickman's task force had finished with Hudson Foods, the story had taken on national and international proportions, with the 'beleaguered' company having to recall 25 million pounds of beef, costing the company its largest customer, Burger King. The resultant fallout devalued Hudson's corporate stock by 35 percent. *The Wall Street Journal* said at the time: 'Hudson's rapid tailspin has stunned some meat industry executives, who blame the record beef recall pushed by the Agriculture Department for breaking the back of Hudson.' 'What happened to Hudson Foods doesn't make sense,' said Patrick Boyle, president of the American Meat Institute.

"[Although] the presence of *E.coli* at the Hudson plant was never proven, the damage had been done. In 1998, Tyson Foods managed to acquire Hudson Foods at a rock bottom price, in a deal described by Leonard Teitlebaum of Merrill Lynch as 'adding beautifully to Tyson's distribution and production system.' *The Wall Street Journal* commented, 'Hudson's brush with Glickman's gang meant the Tyson's buyout bid was an offer the company couldn't refuse.' It is not difficult to see that contrary to Patrick Boyle's comment, the *E.coli* raid made perfect sense."

At about the same time as the Hudson acquisition, events in another part of the world were occurring that also put Tyson in an ideal situation to expand. It was fall, 1997; the first outbreak of avian flu had just occurred in Hong Kong, resulting in the slaughter of two million domestic chickens. Intriguingly, in April of that same year Tyson Foods, together with Thailand's CP, had signed an agreement to build ten giant poultry complexes in China as part of a joint venture with Kerry Holdings Limited, a Hong Kong-based subsidiary of the huge multinational conglomerate, the Kuok Group. This timely agreement solidified Tyson's ability to exponentially expand operations in China and placed Tyson in the powerful position to take over the South China poultry market.[40] To further its stake, in March 2005 Tyson Foods and Fujian Shengnong Group signed an agreement to build the largest chicken processing enterprise in all of southern China.[41]

But Tyson will not be entering the Chinese market unopposed. China has its own entrepreneurs with clear plans of their own for making China's poultry industry the strongest in the world.

New bird flu focus: China and India

Throughout 2004 reports of H5N1 outbreaks among poultry in China were on the rise, but the government denied that any cases of H5N1 had occurred in humans. However, that changed in 2005, and as of December 30, 2005, China had reported to the WHO seven human cases and three deaths scattered across five provinces. Known for hiding the truth from its people, the Chinese government may have been covering up suspected H5N1 deaths for a reason—it may be protecting its commercial poultry and egg industry.

As of 2004, China produced more than 40 percent of the world's eggs. The company largely responsible for the exponential growth is New Hope Ltd., founded in 1982 by the four Liu brothers for a meager investment of US$120. From humble beginnings they worked their way out of poverty and built an empire by selling hog feed to farmers. The Hope Group boasts sales well over US$1billion annually, making the brothers among China's most successful entrepreneurs. In fact, Liu Yongxing and Liu Yonghao, were number one and number two on *Forbes* magazine's "China's 100 Richest Business People" in 2001.[42] In 2005, they were ranked fifth and sixth.[43]

Liu Yongxing envisions revamping and then expanding China's agricultural industry into the most powerful in the world. Knowing his competition and understanding his market, he knows that elimination of the independent farmer is essential to accomplish his goals. In an interview with *Forbes* in November 2005, Liu assessed the problem as one of scale. "A single farmer works on a small farm with his family and might raise a cow or a pig pretty much in the same way that people did 1,000 years ago," he says.

He makes the comparison of pigs born on farms in the U.S. vs. those born in China: Half of the pigs in the U.S. are raised on industrial farms that produce more than 50,000 head per year. In China, 50 percent of pigs are born on farms that raise five or fewer each year. "You can't have a modern industry with that," he says.[44] Having competed for years with Cargill from the U.S. and CP from Thailand, Liu fully understands the steps that need to be taken to implement his plan: Incorporate Tyson-style operations.

Simplifying the process for Liu Yongxing's plan, the transformation to vertically integrated industrial farming is fully backed by the Chinese government. Since the outbreaks began, the minister of agriculture, Du Qinglin, has been advocating for the development of intensive farming, stating, "Bird flu has adversely affected the poultry-raising sector, but in the long haul, it will also prompt a transformation of the [backward] rearing methods, forcing the industry to develop along a healthy and sustainable track."[45]

But the changes will have the same drastic affects on the local Chinese as they are having on Thai and Vietnamese farmers. A story published in the *China Daily* in November 2005 offers an example of the suffering this transition will create. A village farmer, Jiang Lianfu, owned 13,000 healthy, asymptomatic hens that were slaughtered as part of a mass culling of six million birds. Jiang had spent about US$24,700 to establish his henhouse, half with borrowed funds. Instead of paying back his loan in the first year of operation as he had planned, the government paid US$1.20 for each bird culled, or approximately US$15,600, leaving him in debt and without a source of revenue.

As he watched helplessly, armed guards brutally killed his flocks. Jiang told the reporter, "I fed those birds for more than half a year. I treated them like my own children. We just stood there and watched as the birds' necks were wrung."

According to the report, Heishan County, with 15 million hens producing 600 tons of eggs every day, went from being one of Liaoning Province's biggest egg producers to a "virtual chicken ghost town" in less than a week.[46] Culling millions of birds raised by small farmers in areas reported to have an outbreak of H5N1 creates the perfect opportunity for New Hope, positioned with distinct advantages over its international rivals.

In late February 2006, news reports began to shriek of the arrival of bird flu in India. As a "precaution," regional officials killed hundreds of thousands of chickens across the country. But more than bird flu may have been sweeping across the country.

Vertically integrated farming has been entrenched in India for more than 30 years. Founded in 1971, the VH Group (Venkateshwara Hatcheries) is today a $6 billion conglomerate. The largest fully integrated poultry organization in Asia, the VH group is the 5th largest egg producing operation in the world. The group's greatest success has been the use of genetically modified chicken stock from Babcock and Cobb-Vantress. [Notably, Cobb-Vantress, Inc. was formed in 1986 through a joint venture between Tyson Foods, Inc., the owners of the Vantress pedigree line, and the Upjohn Pharmaceutical Company.]

"We are looking at a very difficult future. All of us will have to start again from scratch, and I don't know how many of us will survive," said Ghulam Vhora, a member of an Indian poultry farmers association.[47]

By eliminating the indigenous chickens and the independent farmer, VH Group is positioned to expand the production of its genetically-modified chickens and force the tens of thousands of farmers to work for VH Group. This is similar to what is being done in Thailand by CP Group, in China by the New Hope Group, and in the U.S. by agribusiness conglomerates.

Perhaps Tyson, CP, New Hope, VH, and others have in mind to kill billions of rural chickens, starting in Southeast Asia, China, and India, and then moving across Russia and Eastern Europe, subjugating the independent farmers of those countries to agribusiness. What remains to be seen is the quality of the chickens given to farmers as "replacements" for their free-ranging domestic birds. Quite possibly they will be genetically modified, fast-growing birds created by the world's largest breeders, Aviagen or Tyson's Cobb-Ventress.

If local farmers, and perhaps even governments, fully understood the poultry industry as it exists in the U.S., they might be less willing to sacrifice the local industry and animals to the agribusiness giants.

If we're not willing to settle for junk living,
we certainly shouldn't settle for junk food.
~Sally Edwards, Triathlete, CEO of Heart Zone Training

Chapter 14: Sick Chicks in the U.S.

Starting points:
- Recap of U.S. HPAI virus outbreaks in the last 20 years
- Sick chicks and sick living conditions
- Genetic selection is not the same as genetic modification
- GM crops vs. GM chickens: Is anybody looking for problems?

The killing of domestic flocks has not occurred just overseas. To recap, Highly Pathogenic Avian Influenza (HPAI) viruses are associated with surface antigens H5 or H7. Outbreaks of bird flu in North America that have resulted in the culling of hundreds of millions of birds include the following:

- **1983–5:** An H5N2 outbreak in Pennsylvania that led to the destruction of 17 million birds.
- **February 2004:** An H5N2 outbreak that occurred in Texas, the first outbreak of HPAI in the United States in 20 years. At least 7,000 chickens were destroyed.
- **February 2004:** An H7N3 outbreak that occurred in Fraser Valley, British Columbia. Culling operations eliminated 19 million birds.
- **March 2004:** An H7N2 outbreak in Pocomoke City, Maryland, that led to the culling of more than 500,000 chickens. The Delmarva Peninsula,

which includes parts of Delaware, Maryland, and Virginia, is home to one of the largest concentrations of poultry farms in the U.S.

Culling is the method of choice for suppressing outbreaks of viral epidemics in flocks simply because chickens are considered disposable commodities that can be readily replaced. It takes only 45 days to raise a chick to slaughter weight, so sacrificing the birds is only a short term loss of profits. However, to minimize economic losses, stopgaps have been put in place to protect the large agribusiness companies should an outbreak of HPAI occur in the U.S. For example, when large-scale culling was conducted in the Delmarva Peninsula, the companies that own the birds—such as Tyson, Cargill and Perdue—were required to absorb the first $100,000 of losses, but then the mega-groups were covered by an insurance fund built from the pooled contributions of the major producers. For the Delmarva Peninsula, the fund was in excess of $2.5 million. State governments provide an additional layer of insurance protection for the corporations of up to $5 million, so corporate losses are marginalized by the presence of insurance and government subsidies.

However, culling of stock owned by independent farmers can lead to staggering losses. There are no government programs for individual farm owners, and their birds can be slaughtered by the Department of Agriculture with minimal or no compensation. Since the revenues from chicken production in the Delmarva Peninsula is valued at $1.5 billion annually, whatever losses are incurred by the independent farmers in the region are considered to be "justified" by officials to protect the economic losses of the entire region—and to protect the interests of agribusinesses.[1]

Sick U.S. chicks

Even though all known avian influenza viruses are carried asymptomatically in the intestines of wild birds, domestic chickens can become ill when exposed to influenza viruses. Symptomatic birds display an array of symptoms unique to chickens such as huddling, drop in egg production, tremors, cough, and head tilt.

Other symptoms can include a bloody nasal discharge, facial swelling, and hemorrhages on the shanks. They can shed viruses through saliva, nasal secretions, and excretement when they are under stress. As in humans, there are no pharmaceutical interventions available for the treatment of influenza in birds. The disease can quickly spread through a flock, and if the virus is a highly pathogenic variety the flu can lead to paralysis and rapid death.

Similar to influenza in humans, outbreaks of flu occur among domestic flocks because the birds have compromised immune systems. Becoming ill may have little to do with the "virulence" or "pathogenicity" of the virus and almost everything to do with the state of health of the birds compromised by the established practices of the poultry industry.

The vast majority of broiler chickens in the U.S.—nearly eight billion birds—are raised within the confines of sheds called grower houses. These birds are the most highly confined of all farm animals. A typical grower house can accommodate up to 20,000 chickens so densely packed that each chicken has only 130 square inches of living space; a chicken needs at least 138 square inches of space just to stretch its wings.

Windowless, with forced ventilation to control temperature, grower houses are barren except for floor litter and rows of feeders and drinkers. The high density prevents chickens from practicing many of their normal behaviors including nesting and foraging. Unknown to most, chickens have a carefully regulated social life and a cohesive social structure; extreme crowding stresses the birds and increases the possibility of illness.

Beyond the crushing confinement, conditions within most growers are filthy, forcing birds to be reared in complete squalor. As the chicken excrement accumulates on floors and the bacteria count escalates to break it down, the air becomes polluted with high concentrations of bacteria, fungal spores, and ammonia, all inhaled in dangerous concentrations by both the chickens and their keepers. Ammonia, which is measured in parts per million (ppm), is uncomfortable to humans at 15 ppm and can cause eye irritation, headaches, and a wide range of respiratory problems after a short period. The standard allowable level of ammonia in growers is up to 20 ppm, but in winter levels can exceed 200 parts per million.[2]

For domestic fowl, ammonia can be absorbed through the mucous membranes of the eyes and bronchial tracts, leading to immunosuppression and excess production of mucous. Because birds tend to close their eyes and rub their head against their wings, sustained high levels can cause blindness. Reluctant to move, they may not eat. Congestion in the bronchial tubes destroys the fine hairs in the trachea (cilia) that block the entry of harmful airborne microorganisms, increasing susceptibility to illness. Chickens exposed to 20 ppm of ammonia for 42 days have developed pulmonary congestion, lung hemorrhages, and death.[3] High ammonia levels and closed vents were blamed as the cause of death for thousands of chickens on a farm owned by Tyson Foods in Waldron, Arkansas in 2004.[4]

In October 2001 an Ohio animal rights organization, Mercy for Animals, held a press conference during which it presented the findings of a month-long investigation into the living conditions of hens at the Buckeye Egg Farm and the Daylay Egg Farm, Ohio's two largest egg producers. The investigations uncovered the horrors of how millions of hens are housed in this country. Countless were found sick and injured, suffering from raging eye and sinus infections, pasteurella [bacterial] infections, vitamin deficiencies, and blindness.[5] Several years later, a reporter for the *Baltimore Sun* echoed the findings of Mercy for Animals through a firsthand report of the conditions in the growers after visiting a chicken farm:

> "I recently toured a chicken house and saw firsthand how stressful the environment is. First, if you think chicken houses smell bad from the highway, the air inside is unbearably foul. Particles of manure and feathers hover like a fog while a pall of ammonia stings the eyes. On the ground, a sea of chickens swirl as they seek a little space, decent air, and another snack. After 10 minutes in the chicken house I felt as if I needed an antibiotic."[6]

Beyond stressful living conditions, factory-raised chickens receive a host of vaccines. Beginning on the first day of life, vaccination of chicks begins with a shot for Marek's Disease, a disorder of the nerves and the lymphatic system caused by a herpes virus. An intranasal vaccine for infectious bronchitis is the next shot given during the first week of life, followed by another dose three weeks later. Other routinely administered vaccines include those for Newcastle's disease, fowl pox, and fowl cholera. It stands to reason that the multiple injections of viruses and chemicals in the vaccines—coupled with excessive inhaled ammonia—can lead to compromised immune systems among confined birds. In fact, the presence of increased ammonia alone has been shown to harm the developing immune system in young chicks, increasing the risk of severe vaccine reactions.[7]

At least one particular vaccine has been shown to have a profound effect on the immune system of baby chicks. Recent unpublished experiments indicate that the incidence of vitilego was significantly higher and more severe in chicks that received the vaccine for Marek's Disease compared to those not vaccinated.[8] In humans, vitilego is an acquired autoimmune disorder that results in the loss of pigment resulting in white patches in the skin. In chickens, the vaccine causes brown chickens to turn white. The reason the vaccine triggers the autoimmune response is unknown, but it is thought to be associated with molecular mimicry, a mechanism that has been implicated for a number of vaccine-induced autoimmune disorders in humans.[9] Considering that this vaccine is given in the first day of the chick's life, the evidence that it causes significant immunological disruptions is compelling.

Further compromise: More genetic modification of chickens

The use of selective breeding to ensure the most advantageous attributes in a plant or an animal has been used since 1865, when monk Gregor Mendel proved the existence of inherited traits through his many experiments with pea plants. However, genetic technology of the 21st century has gone far beyond the use of natural selection to attain preferred characteristics. Factory farmed chickens and turkeys are genetically manipulated and bred to grow twice as fast and twice as large as their naturally occurring counterparts.

In the 1950s, it took 84 days to raise a five-pound chicken. Today, due to genetic engineering and growth-producing drugs, a chicken can reach market weight in as little as 45 days. A report from the University of Arkansas's Division of Agriculture puts the rapid growth rate of today's chickens into perspective: "If [a human] grew as fast as a [genetically modified] chicken, you'd weigh 349 pounds at age two."[10]

As for turkeys, *Lancaster Farming* made a similar analogy: "If a seven-pound human baby grew at the same rate that today's turkeys grow, at 18 weeks of age, [the baby] would weigh 1,500 pounds."[11]

While this rapid growth rate is designed to maximize profitability by making harvested muscles larger and lowering feed consumption by limiting days of life, it also exponentially increases the health problems in the birds. A May 1997 *Feedstuffs* article reported that a broiler chicken grows so rapidly that its heart and lungs cannot support the requirements of its body weight, resulting in congestive heart failure and often premature death. The legs of genetically engineered chickens cannot support their unwieldy bodies, resulting in an inability to walk and painful spontaneous hip dislocation.[12]

Genetic modification (GM) has also been applied to the egg-laying capacity of setting hens. Due to the combined genetic and chemical manipulations, a bird is forced to lay an abnormally large number of oversized eggs—up to 250 a year—in contrast to the one or two clutches of about a dozen eggs per clutch laid by her organically-raised relatives. The mechanistic way in which the birds are caged and forced to produce has been likened to "forcing humans to defecate in public."[13] Because the egg industry is now almost completely automated, little is left to nature.

Following the publication of the entire chicken genome in December 2004, a major initiative was launched to identify specific genetic markers for the industry's massive breeding programs. Aviagen, whose poultry breeding brands include Arbor Acres, Ross, and Nicholas Turkeys, is the world's leading poultry breeding company, controlling 35 to 45 percent of the market share for breeding stock worldwide. The agri-giant is studying gene sequences referred to as SNPs (single nucleotide polymorphisms) in an attempt to discover what makes one chicken different from another. Genes are being sought to explain why, given the same feed and management, some chickens grow faster and produce more meat than others. Once identified, the genes can be modified.

Another SNP that researchers are racing to identify is a sequence that would make chickens resistant to influenza viruses. This high-level research, under the direction of researchers Dr. Laurence Tiley from Cambridge University in England and Helen Sang from the Roslin Institute in Scotland, is progressing rapidly. The project involves developing a genetically modified ("transgenic") chicken created to be H5N1-resistant. The idea is that a genetically modified, flu-resistant bird would eliminate the "reservoir" for influenza viruses, making it much more difficult for influenza to jump species and start a pandemic.

The research team is experimenting with three parallel approaches. One method involves inserting a new, active gene into the chicken's DNA that would cause it to manufacture an antiviral protein called Mx. The presence of Mx increases the bird's resistance to influenza strains. A second method involves inserting genes that would inhibit viral replication; without the ability to replicate, a virus cannot spread. The third strategy, similar to the second, involves using RNA molecules as immunological "decoys" that inhibit replication of the virus.[14]

Even if the techniques work as designed, acceptance of these overtly genetically modified chickens may prove to be difficult. Transgenic chickens containing genes derived from viruses will face regulatory hurdles from governments and, hopefully, significant obstacles from both farmers and consumers unwilling to accept these "Franken-chickens" onto their farms and into their diets. Nonetheless, plans for developing this new GM chicken are grandiose, almost beyond comprehension.

Researcher Tiley stated, "Once we have regulatory approval, *we believe it will only take between four and five years to breed enough chickens to replace the entire world population.*" [Emphasis added.][15] To date, it is a little unclear who is funding the development of these birds, but the owner of the GM chickens would conceivably own or control every chicken in the world.

Before the chickens: GM crops

The introduction of genetically modified crops has been dominated and promoted by a handful of corporations. Four companies, Monsanto, Syngenta, Bayer, and Cargill, are responsible for virtually all commercially released GM crops in the world. The reason given by the agri-giants behind the GM technology, under development for nearly 20 years, is to give foods a longer shelf life and easier transportation. For example, inserting a gene from a salmon has created GM tomatoes resistant to cold temperatures. Still under development by Japanese researchers is insertion of a gene from the human liver into rice, enabling the grain to digest pesticides and industrial chemicals.[16]

Corn production in the U.S. is a mega-business. More than 59 percent of the annual U.S. harvest is fed to cattle, hogs, chickens, and other animals. Another 6 percent goes into ethanol production. The breakdown for the rest of the national corn crop usage consists of exports (21 percent), and the manufacture of products such as high-fructose corn syrup for soft drinks (6 percent), cornstarch, and sweeteners (14 percent).[17]

China's Liu Yongxing's intent to expand New Hope's operation from current levels of 700 million broilers to two billion birds in the next three years must be music to the ears of American agribusinesses. Massive expansion of the chicken business will require a massive increase in the amount of corn required to feed the caged birds. "We've been involved with NHG (New Hope Group) for many years now and they are an impressive agricultural force in China," said U.S. Grain Council's senior director of international operations-Asia, Mike Callahan.[18]

Founded in 1960, the U.S. Grain Council is a private, non-profit corporation with programs in more than 80 countries. Its members have one common interest—expanding the export markets for U.S. produced grains. Major participants include the big names in developing genetically modified corn and grains: Monsanto, Monsanto/Corn States Hybrid Service, Syngenta Seeds, Archer Daniels Midland Company, Bayer, and Dow AgroSciences.

Contrary to the claims of GM proponents, GM crops have not been proven to be safe. The regulatory framework for approval of GM foods is based on the principle of "substantial equivalence," an intentionally vague and ill-defined phrase. Because the language is so loosely written, companies developing GM products essentially have a free hand to claim that their transgenic products are "substantially equivalent" to non-GM, natural foods. This is their definition of safe.

To support the illusion of safety when presented to government officials, GM food advocates promote genetic manipulation as a precise technique, deceptively suggesting that a single gene can be inserted into a specific site and that modification will change only one specific characteristic of the food. However, even with the most advanced technology available today, this is not the case. Laboratory technology regarding genetic engineering is crude and imprecise, and the genes being inserted can land anywhere on the host's gene. It is rather like firing a gun loaded with buckshot and hoping one pellet will hit the bull's-eye. Scientists admit they do not fully understand what happens when genes from one organism are inserted into the DNA of another. In addition, the newly inserted "rogue gene" has a tendency to be unstable and drift because it is not firmly anchored into the genetic make up of the host.

Contrary to conventionally believed dogma that one gene governs one particular process, research has shown that genetic material is dynamic and fluid. Genes are constantly changing under the influence of the host's environment or terrain. Geneticists have coined the term "the fluid genome" to encapsulate this paradigm change. In regard to the human genome, scientist Craig Venter explained it this way: "The wonderful diversity of the human species is not hard-wired in our genetic code. Our environments are critical."

The same is true for chickens. If the internal and external environment of domestic fowl is foul, increased genetic manipulation could lead to a plethora of unanticipated consequences. Seeking to insert a foreign gene to change the immune system of an entire chicken can lead to a myriad of unknown results.

The GM products in widest use are soy, cotton, canola, and corn. Of these, a significant furor has been generated around genetically modified corn. GM maize is created by the insertion of a gene called "Bt" because it is taken from a soil-dwelling bacterium, *Bacillus thuringiensis.* The microorganism is capable of producing substances that are toxic to insects. It is thought that by inserting the Bt gene into corn it will also become resistant to insects. Reports of problems abound.

The Institute of Science in Society raised an early red flag after reporting that 12 dairy cows had died in Hesse, Germany, after being exclusively fed a type of GM corn called "GM maize Bt 176™." Other cows had to be slaughtered due to "mysterious illnesses."

In November 2001, the demise of this herd was reported to the Robert Koch Institute in Hesse–responsible for regulating the trials of the GM corn produced by Syngenta. The world's largest seed company, Syngenta controls more than 40 percent of the world's patents on genetically modified grain technologies, including the "Terminator Technology," a method for rendering seeds sterile and forcing farmers to buy new stock each year instead of holding seed in reserve for future planting.[19]

Despite the desperate appeals of the farmer, the Robert Koch Institute did not carry out tests of the GM feed, the surrounding soil, or his dead cows. The minimal investigations were closed by a statement issued two years later by the local district council, proclaiming that the evidence of an association between the GM corn and the death of the cows was "inconclusive" and the cause of the incidents "could not be determined." Tissue samples from the dead cows that had been sent to the University of Göttingen for analysis "vanished in unexplained circumstances."[20]

Barely mentioned in the mainstream press, unlabeled and illegal GM corn contamination has been documented in 27 countries on five continents, and those are only the *recorded* incidents. The worst single contamination incident was of StarLink™ Maize. A GM variety approved only for animal feed, Starlink entered the human food chain in seven countries, Canada, Egypt, Bolivia, Nicaragua, Japan, South Korea, and the U.S.

When the contamination was discovered, the U.S. Environmental Protection Agency (EPA) began to scramble, recalling dozens of products found to be contaminated with StarLink. On September 18, 2000, the *Washington Post* reported that tests ordered by a coalition opposing the biotechnology had found traces of genetic material from StarLink in Kraft's taco shells in grocery stores in Washington, D.C. Several retailers voluntarily recalled corn products from their shelves, but it took the FDA to force the recall of more than 300 GM-contaminated corn products across the country, resulting in losses in excess of US$1billion.

On October 12, 2000, Aventis Crop Science voluntarily withdrew the StarLink registration so it could not be sold or grown in the future. However, three years after the scandal, about one percent of samples tested still contained traces of Starlink. Today the agribusiness giant Syngenta has taken center stage with its production of a new type of GM "terminator technology" corn called GM maize Bt 176™, the same maize that killed the cattle in Germany in 2000.

Once the pollen of GM crops is released into the environment and the seeds are imbedded into the food supply, the consequences are both unpredictable and unknown. In a few more years there may not be many (if any) truly non-GM crops left anywhere in the world. Once GM grains have contaminated the entire planet, the companies that own the patents on the crops will be able to enforce their patent rights, claiming rights to to the land where the crops were grown.

The precedent has already been set. In 2004, Monsanto won a seven-year court battle against a 73-year-old Saskatchewan farmer whose fields had been contaminated by Monsanto's genetically modified plants. The Canadian Supreme Court ruled that the farmer owed Monsanto damages for having Monsanto's patented crops growing illegally in his field. Armed with this legal precedent, the GM seed producers will be in a position to not only own all the farmers of the world, but to own their land too.[21]

Could there be another motive driving agribusiness to create GM, bird-flu resistant chickens? Could it be to create GM chickens that will rapidly achieve market weight only if fed a specific type of GM corn? The idea is not as far-fetched as it might sound. Monsanto's Round-Up Ready GM seeds will sprout and grow only when fertilized by its herbicide, Roundup®. The two are inextricably linked. Perhaps GM chickens and GM corn will be overtly linked, too.

Consider this possible scenario: Every new chick in the world supplanted by a newly created GM chicken—supplied by Aviagen, the biggest supplier of chicks worldwide, or by its biggest competitor, Tyson's Cobb-Vantress. These chicks must be fed GM corn, provided by Monsanto or Syngenta. More than an abject lesson in how a company creates demand for its products, this illustrates how farmers worldwide are targeted to become indentured servants of global agribusiness.

Look deep into nature, and then you
will understand everything better.
~Albert Einstein

Chapter 15: Sick Migratory Birds: Canaries in the Coal Mines

Starting points:
- Agent Orange, still making news after all these years
- Sick sediment makes for sick birds
- Dioxin and influenza viruses: Serious consequences
- Nuclear radiation increases toxic load

Behind the headlines reporting mass culling of flocks around the world and shrieking hysteria about the potential for the H5N1 virus to "jump species" and start the next global pandemic, there is another group of seriously ill birds dying by the thousands—migratory birds. Little mentioned in the news are reports of birds that have been found dead, singularly or en masse, in remote regions across Asia. Many of these birds have tested positive for the H5N1 virus. Is there a viable explanation why free-living birds in nature have become susceptible to this virus? One answer may be in the residuals of war.

The U.S. bombing of Vietnam during that conflict was the most intense episode of aerial blasting known in human history. From 1964 until the war officially ended on August 15, 1973, 6.1 *billion tons* of explosives were detonated throughout Southeast Asia—that's 12,200,000,000,000 pounds of bombs. This represents **roughly** three times as many bombs (by weight) as were dropped in the European and the Pacific theaters combined during World War II, and about 13 times the total tonnage dropped during the Korean War. The heaviest bombing took place in the central region of the country near the 17th parallel, the border between former North and South Vietnam. In the South the so-called "Iron Triangle," a region adjacent to Cambodia near Saigon, was also heavily bombed. Given the prewar Vietnamese population of approximately 32 million, U.S. bombing translates into many hundreds of pounds of explosives per person during the conflict.[1]

In addition to bombs, a 2003 report commissioned by the National Academy of Sciences places the volume of herbicides sprayed between 1961 and 1971 at more than 19 million liters, more than double the official estimate published in 1974. Produced for the Army by several different chemical companies, including T-H Agricultural & Nutrition, Dow Chemical, and Monsanto, the principal chemicals contained a 1:1 mixture of two herbicides introduced in 1947 for control of broad-leaf plants: 2,4-dichloro-phenoxyacetic acid (2,4-D) and 2,4,5-trichlorophenoxyacetic acid (2,4,5-T). The defoliant was later found to be contaminated with a third chemical named 2,3,7,8-TCDD (shortened to TCDD), determined to be the most toxic form of dioxin in the world. Although a colorless liquid, the solution came to be identified by colored stripes painted on the transport barrels. The combo-chemical containing TCDD was known as Agent Orange.[2]

Dioxin is a general term that describes a complex family of more than 400 chemicals that are highly persistent in the environment. It is an unintentional waste product formed during industrial processes that use chlorine. Incineration of plastics, pesticide manufacturing and paper bleaching all result in the production of dioxin. Because chemicals are usually a mixture of toxic and non-toxic compounds, a score for each chemical has been developed called its Toxic Equivalency (TEQ). The TEQ of any chemical is established by comparing it to TCDD, the most toxic form dioxin in the world.

Strictly speaking, this family of chemicals contains 75 chlorinated dioxins, 135 chlorinated furans, and 209 polychlorinated biphenyls (PCBs). Of all these chemicals, 30 have "dioxin-like" toxicity and 17 contribute significantly to the toxicity of mixtures. Because exposures

Agent Orange was not the only horrific chemical used by the U.S. military to douse Southeast Asia during the war in Vietnam. As with Agent Orange, the other chemical names were coined by the military and identified by the color of the stripe painted on the barrel.

Agent Blue, an herbicide composed of a mixture of arsenic compounds, was sprayed on rice paddies and other crops in an attempt to starve the Vietnamese. Since rice is a durable grain, which is difficult to destroy even with conventional explosives and does not burn, the extermination weapon was an herbicide. Agent Blue affects plants by causing them to dry out. Using it on paddies not only destroyed the entire field, but also rendered the land unsuitable for planting in the future.

Agent White, a 4:1 micure of 2,4-D and picloram, was another herbicide used to defoliate possible hiding places of the Vietcong. Picloram can cause central nervous system and liver damage.

Agent Pink, herbicide and defoliant, was composed of 100 percent dioxin.

Agent Purple, chemically named 2,4,5-trichlorophenoxyacetic acid, is a "cousin" to Agent Orange and Agent Pink. It is reported to have had *three times* the concentration of dioxin as Agent Orange.

Although Agent Orange has received the most attention and outrage over the years for the damage it has caused–and continues to cause–veterans, native Vietnamese, and the lands of Southeast Asia, the total amount of dioxin from the combined sprays of other agents remains unknown because records of other agents used are sparse. These known carcinogens do not readily decompose.

usually come as a mixture of toxic and non-toxic compounds, a score is derived by using the International Toxicity Equivalency Factors (TEFs). The TEF of any chemical is also established by comparing it to the toxicity of TCDD.

Recognizing the serious health problems that can occur in the presence of these contaminants, the first Stockholm Convention on Persistent Organic Pollutants (POPs), held in Argentina in May 2001, was convened to address POPs that are (1) intentionally produced, such as pesticides, herbicides, and insecticides; (2) intentionally produced but restricted in use, such as DDT for control of malaria;

and (3) unintentionally produced and released, such as dioxin from herbicides and burning plastics.

An international treaty, which went into force in May 2004, was developed to reduce and eventually eliminate a group of chemicals coined as the "Dirty Dozen" by the United Nations Environmental Program. These 12 chemicals include eight pesticides (aldrin, chlordane, DDT, dieldrin, endrin, heptachlor, mirex, and toxaphene), two industrial chemicals (polychlorinated biphenyls and hexachlorobenzene), and two unintended by-products of chemical production, dioxins and furans.[3]

Of the many concerns voiced over the use of these chemicals, the most ominous is their persistence in the environment. After arriving in the jungles of Vietnam, Agent Orange and other defoliants were mixed with kerosene and diesel fuel before being dispersed by aircraft, by vehicle, and by hand. According to researcher Arthur H. Westing, the sprayings were "frequent and voluminous." As many as 10,000 spraying missions were flown, resulting in dioxin being deposited on more than 15 percent of South Vietnam and a sizable portion of Cambodia and Laos.[4] If deposited into the local water supplies—ponds, lakes, rivers, or streams—dioxin remains in the sediment indefinitely.

In the isolated Aluoi Valley of central Vietnam, very high levels of TCDD were measured in soil samples collected between 1996 and 1999. The valley was the site of a former military base occupied by U.S. Special Forces between 1963 and 1966 and was used as a staging area for Agent Orange missions. The valley is representative of many areas throughout Southeast Asia where large concentrations of TCDD remain in the soil as a result of former military engagements.[5] Research has confirmed that even trace amounts—only two to three parts per trillion (ppt)—are extremely toxic in laboratory animals. More than 30 years later, dioxin continues to be persistent in the food chain, causing potentially deadly contamination of wildlife.[6]

Sick migratory birds

Even though its use as a military defoliant was discontinued in 1971 and one of its components, 2,4,5-T, has been banned in the U.S.

and many other countries, Agent Orange (TCDD) continues to cause health problems in humans and in wildlife due to its lack of biodegradability. A highly persistent chemical, dioxin can take more than 15 years to degrade to half its original concentration. In sub-surface soil it has a great affinity to organic matter and remains largely unchanged, virtually forever.[7] Its persistence in the soil of riverbanks makes it particularly toxic to waterfowl.

Ducks and geese are members of a species group known as the

> In addition to dioxin, five other major pollutants have been found in the sediment of waterways:
> - **Phosphorus and nitrogen compounds** Elevated levels promote the overgrowth of oxygen-consuming algae, leading to the death of fish and other wildlife.
> - **Bulk Organics** A class of hydrocarbons that includes oil and grease.
> - **Polycyclic Aromatic Hydrocarbons (PAH's)** A group of organic chemicals that includes petroleum-based products and by-products.
> - **Metals** These include iron, lead, cadmium, and mercury.
> - **Metalloids** Arsenic
> - **Halogenated Hydrocarbons or Persistent Organic Pollutants (POP's)** A group of chemicals very resistant to decay. Dioxin is in this category.

Anatidae—birds that are ecologically dependent on wetlands for at least some aspect of their annual reproductive cycle. Anatidae species use every conceivable type of wetland across the globe from the high arctic tundra, to freshwater lakes and rivers, to lagoons, mud flats, and the open sea. They also frequent man-made wetlands such as rice fields and other agricultural areas, including irrigation canals. Many of these species migrate between northern breeding grounds and summer nesting areas in Southeast Asia, crisscrossing several continents along the way.

Canadian researchers found that dioxin levels in soil samples throughout different regions of southern Vietnam to be as high as 898 ppt. The most extreme levels of contamination–in the area of Bien Hung Lake–were measured to be *greater than 1.1 million ppt.*[9]

Considering that food for waterfowl–which includes shore grasses, algae, aquatic plants, small fish, tadpoles, and insects–readily absorbs chemicals from the environment, dioxin and other POPs will no doubt accumulate in the fat of birds.[10]

A reasonable assumption can be made that migratory birds have accumulated levels of dioxin in their bodies similar to levels measured in the fat of domestic ducks, where concentrations have ranged from 276 ppt and 331 ppt.[11] The critical point is that dioxin has been shown to disrupt the immune system at concentrations as low as 1.0 ppt. This is the equivalent of a single drop of liquid placed in the center car of a ten-kilometer (6.2 miles) cargo train.[11] Even though this amount seems inconsequentially small, a tiny drop can cause substantial health problems in humans and birds alike.

Unfortunately, little is known about the full impact of chemicals on wildlife, as few measurements have been taken, making it difficult to assess the chemical ramifications in migratory birds. Testing thousands of live, wild birds is impractical, and few dead birds are available to test. Most often, birds die in isolation and scavengers consume the carcasses within days. In addition, the chemical analyses required to determine if, indeed, a bird's death was due to a poison are costly and difficult to perform; therefore, they are seldom carried out. Making the assessment even more difficult is the fact that toxicity differences among chemicals vary between species, sometimes by a factor of 10 or more. Baseline toxicities of individual chemicals in wild birds, not to mention TEQs of combined chemicals, are completely unknown.

Although exact concentrations are unknown, what *is* known, is that a definite link exists between dioxin exposure and the effect of influenza viruses on the immune system. This connection has been studied in experimental animals in the laboratory.

Dioxin combined with influenza viruses: Serious consequences

Studies conducted over the past 25 years have established that the immune system can be compromised by infinitesimally small amounts of TCDD. Although the mechanisms are not well understood, the adverse effect most consistently reported in toxicology literature is TCDD's ability to suppress the function of white blood cells (T-lymphocytes), essential for fighting infection. Studies confirm that both humans and birds are much more likely to have a deadly result when confronted with an influenza A virus if they have also been exposed to dioxin.

TCDD suppresses the activity of cytotoxic lymphocytes (CTLs), specialized white blood cells that eliminate viruses and bacteria. Two primary types of "killer" white blood cells exist—natural killer cells (NK) and CD8+ cells. Both vigilantly circulate through the blood destroying unwanted particles as they are found. NK and CD8+ cells do their work by releasing granules that cause infected cells to break apart; hence, the virus "dies" because it cannot replicate. After the cell has been destroyed, the NK and CD8+ cells move on to snuff out more virus-containing cells. It is believed that without fully functioning CTLs, the host's defenses can become overwhelmed by the replicating germs, even leading to death.

The body is very conservative in its use of vital resources. In a healthy state, only a minimal number of NK and CD8+ cells are in circulation, acting as sentinels. However, if the number of viral particles detected is on the rise, elimination calls for the rapid increase in the number of NK and CD8+ cells in circulation. Once activated, the CTL cells release proteins called cytokines, chemical messengers that recruit dozens of other specialized white blood cells that are necessary to eliminate the virus. Cytokines are responsible for causing acute reactions in the body including pain, fever, and inflammation. It is this ramping-up within the immune system that produces the readily recognized symptoms of "the flu."

"Influenza severity" has been correlated with cytokine production. In other words, the more cytokines that are released in the presence of an influenza virus, the more serious the infection and the more potentially deadly the outcome. There are many different cytokines involved in this complex process, but the two that are relevant to this discussion are IL-12 (interleukin 12) and IFNγ (interferon-gamma). Cytokine IL-12 plays the key role in coordinating the efforts of the entire immune system's campaign against a virus, while IFNγ facilitates the destruction of cells that contain replicating viruses.

Research has clearly demonstrated that NK and CD8+ cells are exquisitely sensitive to extremely small concentrations of TCDD. In 2000, studies showed that if mice had been subjected to 100-1000 ppt of TCDD prior to being exposed to common influenza A viruses, the number of mice that died was significantly higher than the number of control mice that were not pre-exposed to this dioxin.[12] In an earlier study, Burleson (1996) determined that giving mice a mere 10 ppt of TCDD one week before they were exposed to influenza A viruses, *the mortality rate among the mice doubled.* Researchers noted that this was the "smallest toxic dose ever demonstrated" to inhibit the ability of the immune system to ward off the flu.[13]

Even though the mechanism for how dioxins disrupt the immune system is not completely understood, there is overwhelming evidence that exposure to TCDD significantly inhibits the host's ability to resist influenza. First, in the presence of dioxin the "ramping-up" response doesn't occur. The needed killer white blood cells are not produced, and the functional capacity of the ones in circulation is significantly compromised. Second, TCDD causes a disruption in the activity of cytokines in lung tissue, suppressing the production of cytokine IL-12. Without IL-12, other white blood cells are not recruited to aid in the elimination of the virus. At the same time, TCDD increases the levels of IFNγ by more than 10-fold. Rampant production of IFNγ leads to massive inflammation, not only killing infected cells, but also causing extreme damage to normal lung cells in the area of the infection. The runaway hyper-production of IFNγ and other inflammatory cytokines is called a cytokine storm. It is the pressure of a cytokine storm that increases the mortality among TCDD-exposed mice.[14]

It has long been presumed that death due to influenza is a

result of rampant proliferation of viruses that overwhelm the capacity of the body to respond. In other words, the immune system is so compromised by the virus that its massive replication kills the host.

Interestingly, studies have determined that, particularly when dioxin is involved, *this is not the case.* A study done by Luebke (2002) examined fluid extracted directly from the lungs of deceased mice. The results proved that the increased mortality seen in TCDD-exposed mice was due to the intense inflammatory action of dioxin. In other words, the *combination of influenza viruses and dioxin caused so much inflammation in the lungs*—due to a massive cytokine storm—that normal lung tissue was destroyed, leading to death of the mice.[15]

Researchers have discovered that some influenza viruses are definitely capable of causing a more intense inflammatory response than others. The same intense reactions observed in the lungs of dioxin-laden mice that are infected with influenza have been observed in human lung cells artificially infected with H5N1 in the laboratory. In a study conducted by Chan, et al. in November 2005, H5N1 viral subtypes isolated from Vietnamese patients mixed with human lung tissue cells induced "unusually high levels of pro-inflammatory cytokines," much higher than the inflammatory cascade produced by "garden variety" seasonal influenza viruses.[16]

Malik Peris, professor of microbiology at Hong Kong University and part of the Chan research team, discussed the results in an interview with *The Standard,* a Chinese business newspaper: "We found that infection with H5N1 viruses led to the production of 10 times higher levels of cytokines in human cells than normal human flu viruses." Peiris went on to say, "The reason H5N1 virus behaves like this is still being investigated." In other words, the reason for this observation is unknown.[17]

A thought-provoking question to be raised regarding the Chan study relates to the fact that the human lung tissue used for the research was obtained from 13 patients, ranging in age from 46 to 77 years, who were undergoing surgery at Grantham Hospital, Hong Kong, for the removal of lung tumors. The cells, selected from sections of tissue that did not contain tumor cells, were subjected to solutions to separate them into a single layer. Is it possible that the cells used in the lab contained traces of dioxin? It is a reasonable assumption that these patients—living in Hong Kong and suffering from lung cancer—may have been exposed to cancer-causing dioxin.

Several lines of evidence indicate that most, if not all, biologic responses caused by dioxin occur after it binds tightly to a specific cellular protein termed "AhR," found in all tissues and all species. After binding occurs, the AhR-dioxin complex moves into the nucleus of the cell, interacts with specific binding sites, and changes the function of genes. Detecting the presence of dioxin that has already been integrated into a cell requires very sensitive assays. The method, described as the only way to accurately detect the presence of dioxin in cells, uses techniques borrowed from modern molecular biology. Seventeen different toxic dioxin and furan compounds can be detected in concentrations as small as 0.2 parts per trillion.[18] Because the tests are very expensive, it is unlikely that the experimental human lung cells were tested for the presence of dioxin prior to being exposed to H5N1. (It is known that H5N1 and dioxin can both induce a cytokine storm in lung tissue.) Could the combination of the two determine whether bird flu—in humans or in birds—will have a fatal outcome? Further study is needed to fully evaluate the relationship between human lung tissue, H5N1, and dioxin. Perhaps the missing link—why many humans and birds have been exposed to H5N1 but few have died—has to do with the toxic load of dioxin in their lungs.

Migratory bird contamination: From chemicals to nuclear waste

The largest lake in China, Qinghai Lake, covers an area of nearly 1,800 square miles (4,583 square kilometers) and is an important rendezvous site for migratory birds traveling from Southeast Asia to the Central Asian winter breeding grounds. The lake sits at an altitude of 10,712 feet (3,266 meters) and is also called "Lake Kokonor" in Mongolian, meaning "blue lake," reflecting the extraordinary turquoise blue hues of the water. On the Tibetan end of the lake, it is also called "Lake Tso Ngonpo." Near the center of the lake is a peninsula referred to as "Bird Island," a nature preserve, which covers more than 135,000 square acres (54,200 sq. ha.)

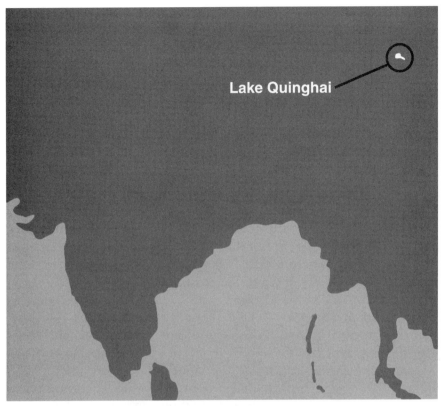

Location of Qinghai Lake in the NE
part of China's Qinghai-Tibet Plateau
(map reproduced with permission)

Lake Kokonor, known for more than 8,000 years for its fresh water, is now considered to be brackish. Its size has been diminishing an average of five inches (12.7 centimeters) per year. This is attributed to the present rate of evaporation and to modern agriculture's over-utilization of the lake's water, both of which far exceed the amount that can be replenished by local rainfall and run- off.

The lake is bustling with bird activity throughout most of the year. Estimates vary, but it is thought that at any one time, more than 300,000 fowl can be wafting across its waters. In all, at least 189 species of birds have been recorded around the lake including several globally threatened species such as the black-necked crane. The largest contingent spends its time on Bird Island during the nesting season (May–August), and many more species arrive as part of their seasonal migration (March–May and August–November). Based on its international importance, Bird Island has been designated as a Ramsar Site, a treaty-protected international wetland area.[19]

Unfortunately, when migratory birds arrive at this traditional resting point they find conditions on Bird Island have deteriorated dramatically in recent years. Poorly representative of a "nature preserve," the lake's waters are anything but pristine. On the north side is a labor camp that is part of the extensive Chinese gulag. The sandy eastern shores are home to the Haiyan nuclear weapons facility called the "Ninth Academy," or "Factory 221." This has been the site of China's main nuclear research and production since the 1960s. The compound, also known as the "Northwest Nuclear Weapons Research and Design Academy," houses the design facility that has carried out non-nuclear explosions and many other nuclear weapons-related activities over the last 40 years.

Radioactive waste generated during weapons production was dumped into the lake from the Research Academy well into the 1980s. All along, the Chinese government has staunchly rejected accusations of environmental damage at the site and, more ominously, retorted that "no one at the base ever died of radiation poisoning." Without

Historical/Political Side Note:

The significance of placing nuclear weapons on the Tibetan plateau is also critical to understanding historical and current geo-political relationships. In 1964, when China conducted its first nuclear blast, India began its nuclear program. The prospect of being faced with superior conventional nuclear forces on the Tibetan plateau exacerbated India's unease. India's sense of vulnerability increased dramatically with China's military alliance with Pakistan. Today, India and Pakistan are both involved in nuclear weapons production.

data, there has been no mechanism to assess the cumulative amount of radioactive pollution released into the rivers, pastures, and surrounding lakes.[20]

China finally came clean in 1995 and not only admitted to the existence of a nuclear dump at the Ninth Academy site, but also confessed that an unknown quantity of radioactive material in the forms of "liquid slurry, gases, solid waste, and wastes from fuel concentration reprocesses" had been released throughout the area. The most unsettling disclosure was that this toxic cocktail had been discharged continually since the 1960s into shallow, unlined landfills seeping into the groundwater that flows into Lake Kokonor.

Tibetans living near the Ninth Academy informed the Tibetan Government-in-Exile in 1996 that Chinese security personnel secretly guarded the Ninth Academy area around the clock. A functioning direct railway connects the facility with Lake Kokonor, and nuclear waste experts believe that radioactive waste continues to be dumped directly into the lake.[21]

The Tibetan Plateau is the planet's largest and highest plateau. It is home to the 14 highest peaks in the world, all over 26,000 feet (8,000 meters). The 10 major rivers flowing from its glaciers sustain 85 percent of Asia's population—47 percent of the world's population. With Asia so heavily dependent upon Tibet for its water, nuclear-related pollutants dumped into its lakes have massive implications for nations downstream. Lake Kokonor is a watershed that eventually becomes the Yellow River, one of the two largest rivers in all of China.

A survey completed in 1994 found that only 32 percent of China's river water met the national standards for drinking water. The health of these water systems determines the survival of most inhabitants—human, animal, and bird—throughout China and Southeast Asia.[22]

Although specific research documenting the effects of nuclear contamination on birds breeding on Bird Island has either not been done or is highly classified, evaluation of the state of waterfowl exposed to nuclear wastes in the U.S. can give insight into the health risks posed to migratory birds by radiation-contaminated waters in China and Southeast Asia.

For more than 40 years, the U.S. government produced plutonium for nuclear weapons at the Hanford Site in south central Washington State. From World War II until the early 1970s, Hanford released radioactive elements and other harmful materials directly into the Columbia River. The river downstream from Hanford held the distinction for many years as the most radioactive waterway in the United States. Seasonal ducks and geese that nested or fed along the Columbia became so highly contaminated with radiation that the consumption of a one-half pound serving of the most contaminated duck meat would have delivered four times the dose of radiation to the consumer's bones allowed by *annual* limits.[23]

In 1988, experiments were conducted in Southeastern Idaho to identify the level of radioactive accumulation in mallard ducks that had been living for at least five months on a lake designated as a radioactive waste disposal site. When the birds were sacrificed, radioactive particles were found in their bones, feathers, and livers. The highest concentrations were found in the gastrointestinal tract—concentrations that were similar to the amounts identified in the vegetation, insects, and sediments within the ponds.

Like dioxin and other POPs, radiation—in the form of radionu-clides—can pass up the food chain from sediments into wild birds. Weeds and other algae have a remarkable capacity to concentrate radionuclides up to 100,000 times the levels found in the water. Resident fish and amphibians collect higher concentrations through skin absorption and through consumption of aquatic grasses and insects.[24] There can be little doubt that the level of radioactive contamination in ducks and geese that spend time on Lake Kokonor and the rivers it feeds would be the same or greater than those found in U.S. waterfowl.

Couple this with the toxic chemicals the birds consume during the summer in Southeast Asia prior to their arrival at the Tibetan lake, and it is no wonder that the birds are sick. The actual cause of death of the huge number of birds at Lake Kokonor is officially unknown. However, compelling evidence suggests they may have died from a combination of nuclear waste exposure and chemical contamination.

Migratory birds: NOT spreading H5N1

Several events have been reported involving mass mortalities of large flocks of migratory birds. In August 2005, Mongolia reported the death of some 90 wild birds at two different lakes in separate parts of the country. Between May and July 2005, officials reported that more than 6,000 dead birds were found around Lake Kokonor, with many testing positive for H5N1.

Receiving the most media attention was the death of 178 bar-headed geese. These large, powerful birds are known to fly expansive distances, soaring over the Himalayas during their migration from Southeast Asia and parts of Northern India on their way to Central Asia. This is normal for this species, and yet, one report stated, "It is believed that migrating bar-headed geese *were exhausted on arrival* at Qinghai Lake and fell easy prey to the H5N1 flu virus."[25] Not only does this explanation sound implausible for the simultaneous deaths of these sturdy birds, but it also lacks scientific credibility.

Because they travel over great distances and a few dead birds have tested positive for the H5N1 virus, migratory birds have been blamed as the vector for transmitting the virus far and wide. But there are flagrant holes in this accusation. First, little is actually known about the precise migration routes of most waterfowl. Many do not follow the generally accepted paths called flyways; many spend their non-breeding periods soaring throughout two or more flyways. In addition, the flyway areas share considerable overlap, especially throughout the northern latitudes where the birds breed. Despite aggressive efforts undertaken by many groups to identify migratory patterns of bird species, very few tagged birds have ever been recovered. Without the evidence of actual birds, a comprehensive analysis of the migratory pathways, timing of movements, and areas of greatest concentration is precluded.[26] Most importantly, outbreaks have not coincided with arrival of the migratory birds to specific areas.

To blame the scattered H5N1 outbreaks that have occurred across Asia, Turkey, and Eastern Europe on migratory birds when so little is actually known about their migration patterns is nothing more than an *uneducated* guess. Keep in mind that most avian influenza viruses exist in the intestines of wild birds symbiotically and asymptomatically. As stated succinctly by author Wendy Orent in *The LA Times,* "Sick birds don't fly far and dead birds don't fly at all."[27]

Despite little evidence to indicate that wild birds are the source of HPAI outbreaks, in October 2005, government officials throughout Britain, Russia, Ukraine, Romania, and Turkey shockingly asked hunters to shoot down as many incoming ducks and geese as possible so they could be tested for the H5N1 virus.[28] It would be humorous if it were not so serious. The WHO had the foresight to declare that wild birds should not be culled; experts warned that some migratory species are rare and their extinction could have far-reaching ecological consequences.[29] Thankfully, *someone* was thinking.

Scientific confirmation that H5N1 is not spread by migratory birds continues to mount. Flocks of migratory birds returned to Europe in the spring of 2006 from Africa without any evidence of the virus. Bird flu specialist with Wetlands International, Ward Hagemeijer, confirmed that, contrary to what people had expected, the virus was not being spread by wild birds. More than 7,500 samples were collected from birds in Africa during the preceding winter and H5N1 was not detected *in a single wild bird.* In Europe, only a few cases were detected in wild birds during the height of the migration north, negating the theory of migratory birds as the vector for spreading the flu.[30]

In spite of the evidence, testing wild birds continues. In May 2006, the search for the first wild bird carrying H5N1 into North America began on a stretch of coastal salt marsh on the outskirts of Anchorage, Alaska.[31] Washington state biologists planned tests for 2,500 wild birds in July 2006 as part of the national effort to detect bird flu when it enters the continental U.S. The Department of Fish and Wildlife stated it would focus on several species of migratory shorebirds and waterfowl that were "most likely to interact with Asian migratory birds in the Arctic."[32] At the cost of tens of millions of dollars—here and abroad—these activities may be an implementation of Step 5 in the New Playbook: "Give people something to do."

Creating a model that blames wild birds for spreading the virus to domestic chickens and then on to humans is simply a convenience. Deaths of migratory birds occurring at about the same time or in the same vicinity as outbreaks and deaths among domestic birds do not mean that the events are related. In the vaccine world, the defining phrase for this apparent connection is "temporal association does not prove causality," meaning, when two events occur at nearly the same time, one doesn't necessarily cause the other. In other words, even though H5N1 has been detected in sick chicks and dead migratory birds in close proximity to each other, one didn't necessarily infect the other.

More likely, the horrific living conditions of industrially raised chickens and the exposure of wild birds to substantial environmental toxicities have suppressed the immune system of both sets of birds. During long migrations, the birds undergo stressful conditions that utilize energy reserves. Burning fat stores will mobilize the chemicals that are stored in fat, creating acute poisoning of the birds. The combination of environmental toxicities—dioxin, nuclear radiation, and other POPs, with H5N1—has led to deadly inflammation in the tissues in both types of fowl, leading to their demise. Wild birds and domestic chickens may well be described as the *victims* of bird flu, not the *vectors,* and H5N1 is a *contributing factor* to the demise of birds loaded with toxicities rather than the *causative* factor. What is happening to the birds around the world should be serving as a resounding wake-up call for the foul condition of planet Earth.

In fact, this connection has been proven in at least one instance. Pesticide application has been increasing over the last 50 years in Latin and South America and has caused significant problems for migratory birds. In 1994, 4,100 Swainson hawks were found dead in four separate locations, which later proved to be caused by monocrotophos. Banned in the U.S. in 1985, this pesticide is known to be dangerous to mammals and birds even though it remains the third most used pesticide in Central and South America.[33]

The FAO has reported, "There remains a body of data that is missing on the collection and detection of HPAI viruses from wild birds."[34] Clearly, the FAO's "missing data" is the impact of environmental chemicals and nuclear wastes on migratory birds, increasing their risk of a terminal outcome in the presence of influenza viruses, including H5N1.

195

Sickness comes on horseback, but goes away on foot.
~William C. Hazlitt, English Writer (1778-1830)

Chapter 16: Sick Humans

Starting points:
- Dioxin in food
- Effects of dioxin and POPs on the immune system
- Sick humans in Vietnam, China, and Turkey: The connection

Experiments with mice have demonstrated that the immune system is exceedingly sensitive to the effects of TCDD and other dioxin-like chemicals. Deaths from "garden variety influenza" occurred due to extreme inflammation in the lungs when the virus was combined with tiny doses of dioxin. The chemical suppresses the effectiveness of white blood cells that eliminate viruses, (NK and CD8+ cells), leaving the immune system vulnerable. Importantly, mice and humans have similar degrees of sensitivity to dioxin-influenza combinations.

A study published in the September 29, 2005, edition of the *New England Journal of Medicine* summarized the features of a human H5N1 infection. The cluster of symptoms observed included fever, cough, shortness of breath, elevated liver enzymes, pulmonary infiltrates (pneumonia), and lymphopenia (low white blood cell count). Upper respiratory tract symptoms were rarely present. All of these symptoms are similar to those observed in TCDD-laden mice that are exposed to benign, low-pathogenic influenza viruses.[1]

Dioxins are perhaps the most studied of all chemicals, as there are more than 5,000 published scientific papers on the effects of TCDD, with many hundreds specifically identifying its danger to human health. Despite the voluminous documentation of its hazards, the party line spewed by the EPA and the chemical industry for more than 20 years has been that low levels of dioxin pose no health problems. In fact, U.S. Assistant Surgeon General Vernon N. Houk, MD, who was also the top official at the CDC in 1992, completely downplayed the health threat of dioxin. Amazingly, he even stated that the government should "relax somewhat the amount of dioxin it says humans can safely ingest."[2]

Fortunately, time and science have prevailed. On January 19, 2001, the National Institutes of Environmental Health Sciences added TCDD to the list of substances known to be human carcinogens. The dioxin found in Agent Orange has been associated with blood cancers—non-Hodgkin's lymphoma, Hodgkin's disease and chronic lymphocytic leukemia (CLL)—and soft tissue sarcomas.[3]

In addition to the medically-confirmed and government-recognized cancers, the Veteran's Administration offers the following list of conditions reportedly associated with exposure to Agent Orange: prostate cancer, respiratory cancers, multiple myeloma, type II diabetes, peripheral neuropathy, and spina bifida in children of exposed veterans.[4]

Studies attempting to prove these connections among American veterans have had mixed results, perhaps because too much time had lapsed between the exposures and the research. The biological half-life of TCDD in humans without ongoing exposure is thought to be 5.8 to 14.1 years. Testing veterans 30 years after exposure may show little trace of the original chemical.[5]

Beyond looking at Americans who were exposed during the war, some research has been done among Vietnamese who had substantially higher exposures overall, and continue to have high daily exposures of dioxin through their contaminated soil and food. In a study published in April 2003, lead researcher Jeanne Mager Stellman of Columbia University used overlooked pilot flight logs—documenting more than 10,000 spraying missions—to construct the most sophisticated computerized maps ever produced of herbicide spraying in Vietnam. Stellman's team was able recreate the flight paths, combine them with the amount and type of agents delivered, and superimpose the patterns on the known location of troops and the Vietnamese populations. Using census data for 20,000 Vietnam villages, Stellman's study corroborated that more than 3,100 towns were sprayed directly, affecting between two million and four million people.[6] More than 30 years after the end of the spraying, these highly persistent chemicals are still affecting the Vietnamese.

One of the few studies undertaken on the local population was completed in 1986. Researchers J. Constable and Hoang Trong Quynh collected samples of human fat from 120 randomly selected southern Vietnamese citizens who had entered a hospital in Ho Chi Minh City (formerly Saigon) for a variety of surgical operations. Sent to laboratories in the U.S., Canada, Sweden, and Germany for analysis, the fat samples revealed that 81 percent of the patients had dioxin in their tissues above accepted "background levels" of 2–3 ppt, a unit of measure that is also expressed as nanograms per kilogram of body weight, or ng/kg.[7]

Several years later, between 1991 and 1992, a similar study examined pooled blood collected from patients throughout southern Vietnam. The results documented that people living throughout the country continued to show elevated TCDD levels, up to 33 ppt, more than 10 times higher than average acceptable background levels for humans.[8]

A more recent study by Schecter (2003) demonstrated similar findings. Blood samples from more than 3,200 persons were collected in both southern and northern Vietnam and analyzed for more than 160 different dioxins and dioxin-like chemicals. Researchers were astonished to discover that some Vietnamese had extremely high concentrations of dioxins in their bodies. Nearly 95 percent of the 43 people tested from Bien Hoa City, a large metropolitan area in southern Vietnam, had TCDD levels as high as *413 ppt* in their blood. Strikingly, this city has developed over the grounds of a former U.S. air base that staged hundreds of Agent Orange spraying missions. Bien Hoa City is approximately 20 miles north of Ho Chi Minh City, and is one of many cities in the Mekong Delta considered to be "dioxin hot spots" due to their high concentrations of residual chemicals.

The Mekong Delta is the region in Southeast Vietnam where the Mekong River empties into the sea. One of the great rivers of Asia, the Mekong ranks as the twelfth longest river in the world and sixth in terms of mean annual discharge. It begins in the Tanghla Shan Mountains, on the northeast rim of the great Tibetan Plateau, and flows for more than 2,500 miles (4,160 km) through or along the borders of six countries: China, Burma, Laos, Thailand, Cambodia, and Vietnam.

Absent ongoing aerial spraying, dioxin's primary route for entering the body is through food. Research was undertaken in 2002 to test the levels of dioxin and POPs in animals raised for consumption in the Bien Hoa City region. A total of 16 different food samples were collected from local markets around Bien Hung Lake and from farms near the air base where Agent Orange had been stored. Samples included the most commonly consumed meats: free-ranging and cooped chickens, free-ranging ducks, pork, beef, fish, and a toad. Because duck fat is a delicacy in Vietnam, fat that remained attached to the flesh of samples was also tested. All samples were frozen and shipped to a state-of-the-art diagnostic laboratory in Hamburg, Germany, for analysis of persistent organic pollutants (POPs), including dioxins, dibenzofurans, and PCBs.

The preliminary results were startling. Three of the specimens contained dioxin levels that were so extraordinarily high they were sent to a second, independent laboratory for additional analysis. The second lab confirmed the disturbing results.

In the final report, dioxin and other chemical contaminants were detected in all 16 food samples. The selection that stood out as "markedly elevated" was the fat of ducks, with levels ranging between 276 ppt and 331 ppt wet weight. When the TEQ score—a sum of all toxic chemicals measured—was tabulated for the duck fat, the score ranged from 536 ppt to 550 ppt. To put these elevated levels in perspective, the usual dioxin level found in food is **less than 0.1 ppt.**[9]

Among the extremely toxic foods measured at 65 ppt, was the Channa striata (snakehead fish). This fish survives the dry season by burrowing into the mud at the bottom of lakes and streams, subsisting on its own stored body fat. Reflecting the contamination of local soil, the chemicals found in free-ranging chickens ranged from 15 ppt in the meat and up to 74 ppt in the fat. Meat from caged chickens was found to have relatively low concentrations of dioxins—but these animals have their own set of problems, as discussed previously. The most likely exposure for industrially raised birds is through water and feed.

Because areas of Laos and Cambodia were also exposed to Agent Orange between 1962 and 1971 , 28 food samples consisting of meat, fish, and dairy products were collected from sprayed areas in these countries and compared with samples from non-sprayed areas. Fish samples from the Agent Orange-sprayed area had nearly 32 percent more dioxin than fish from non-sprayed areas, suggesting that the sediment in the soil of Laos remains toxic and the chemical is still being incorporated into the food chain.[10]

With such high levels of chemicals found in chickens and ducks, it should be no surprise that equally high levels of dioxins and other POPs have been discovered in their eggs. A 2005 study sponsored by the International POPs Elimination Network (IPEN) tested eggs of free-range chickens from 20 different locations and 17 countries: Belarus, Bulgaria, Czech Republic, Egypt, India, Kenya, Mexico, Mozambique, Pakistan, Philippines, Russia, Senegal, Slovakia, Tanzania, Turkey, Uruguay, and the U.S. Chicken eggs were chosen because they are a common food and the fat in their yolks is the repository for chemicals. Further, the diet of backyard and free-range hens—worms, insects, grasses, and other small organisms—makes eggs a useful indicator of overall local environmental contamination.[11]

The results were eye-opening and highly disturbing. The lowest levels of dioxins measured in eggs from these 17 developing countries were *more than twice the concentration* of dioxin in eggs sampled from Europe and North America. In fact, 70 percent of the samples exceeded the 2002 European Union (EU) limit for dioxins in eggs, which is 0.75 ppt. The highest levels, found in the eggs of chickens raised near a toxic waste dump in Russia, reached 44.69 ppt.

Although eggs from Vietnam, Cambodia, and Thailand were not specifically tested in this survey, levels measured in surrounding countries are likely to be representative. Dioxin measurements in eggs from the Philippines were 9.68 ppt. In Lucknow, northern India, and in Eloor, southern India, levels were 19.80 ppt and 13.91 ppt, respectively.[12] The concentrations are directly proportional to the amount of toxicity in the local environments. Studies tracing the movement of POPs from soil to organisms to chickens, and from chickens to their eggs have found that the chemical concentration in farmland and riverbank sediment correlates with concentrations found in eggs.[13]

The high doses of deadly dioxins are being consumed daily by the people of Vietnam. The potential for adverse health effects resulting from exposure to dioxin-laden compounds can be determined by using tables compiled through the Agency for Toxic Substances and Disease Register (ATSDR). This federal agency, which is part of HHS, is responsible for preventing or reducing the harmful effects that hazardous substances can have on health. Using a unit of measure called minimal risk levels (MRLs), ATSDR establishes the dose below which adverse health effects are not expected to occur (so-called "safe" dose).

Even though it sounds like a reasonable measure, the MRL is not the value used by the EPA to predict the harmful effects of a chemical. Another unit, called the "oral reference dose" (RfD), has been established by the EPA. By definition, the RfD is "an *estimate* of a daily exposure in humans that *is likely* to be without an *appreciable* risk of deleterious (harmful) effects *during a lifetime.*" [Emphasis added.] The EPA admits that risks of environmental exposure "cannot be scientifically distinguished from an estimate."[14] In other words, the RfD is simply a "guess" as to the level that can cause harm.

The WHO has developed a measure for dioxin risk related to the Tolerable Daily Intake (TDI). Endorsed by international committees, the TDI estimates the amount of a chemical—or a mix of chemicals —that, even if ingested every day over a lifetime, is not thought to be harmful to human health. For dioxin, the TDI is 0.010 ppt/day (10 pg per day). Adverse effects from dioxins have been documented at levels much lower than the allowed TDI. For example, infants in the Netherlands whose mothers had been exposed to an average daily dose of dioxin of 3 pg per day showed slight neurological effects, hormonal changes and suppressed immune functions (Huisman 1995). Many other studies have shown similar results. Amazingly, the WHO has found it acceptable to allow the TDI for dioxin to remain as high as 10 pg per day because it didn't consider these subtle effects "adverse enough to cause concern."[15]

The ongoing exposure to dioxin may very well be the reason that southern Vietnam has had the largest number of human bird flu deaths to date. Between December 26, 2003, and June 16, 2006, a total of 227 confirmed human cases of avian influenza (H5N1) have occurred worldwide. Of 129 deaths reported in nine countries, Vietnam has suffered 43 deaths. These could be associated with high concentrations of dioxin.

Even though the effects of low-level, continuous exposure to dioxin have not been clearly established in humans, studies in experimental animals can be used as a comparison. Because science has long established that mice have biochemical profiles similar to humans, the effects of dioxin observed in mice—increased inflammation and death when dioxin and influenza commingle in the lungs—would likely be consistent with effects in humans.

The citizens of southern Vietnam are not only consuming dioxin-laden foods; many have continuous exposures from the soil where they live. There is a disquieting overlap between maps documenting the spraying of Agent Orange during the war and outbreaks of H5N1 in birds and humans. The maps, provided through the U.S. Army and by the former executive director of the New Jersey Agent Orange Commission, Bill Lewis, demonstrate a striking overlap with a map constructed by the FAO. The greatest numbers of poultry and humans H5N1 infections are in the same areas as the heaviest sprayings of Agent Orange.

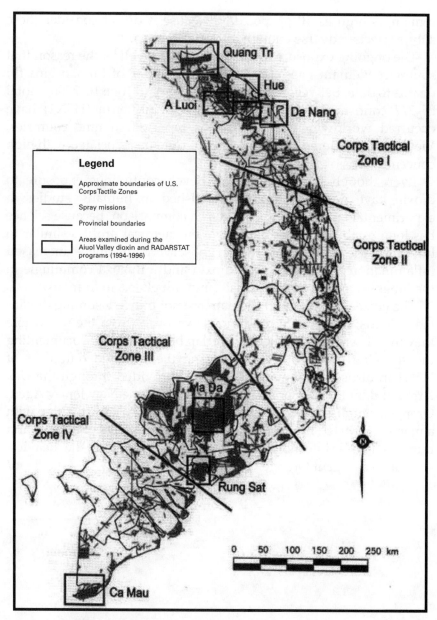

Aerial herbicide spray missions in southern Vietnam, 1965 to 1971.
(Source: U.S. Dept. of the Army).

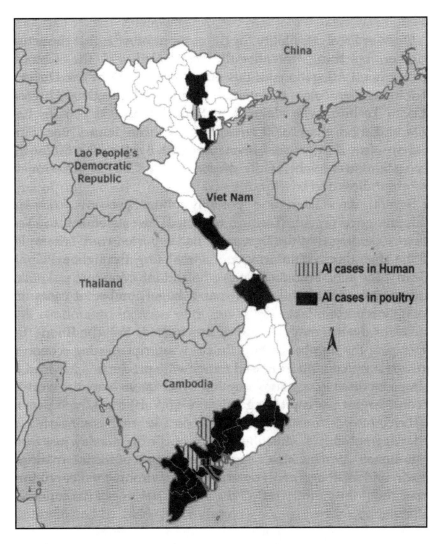

Provinces reporting avian influenza outbreaks in poultry and humans in Vietnam since December 2004 (as of 27 January 2005)

Reproduced with permission from the Food and Agriculture Organizations of the United Nations

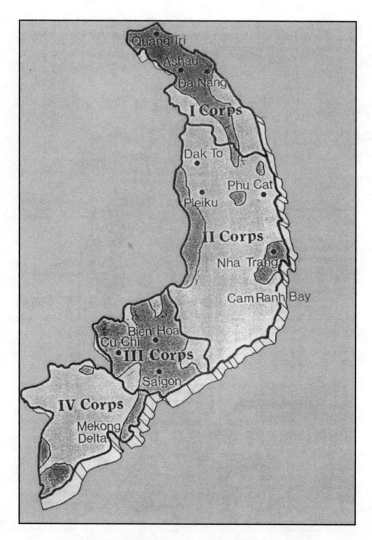

This map represents only fixed-wing aircraft spraying of Agent Orange and does not include helicopter spraying of perimeters or other spray methods. The III Corps area recieved the heaviest concentrations of spraying, followed by I Corps, II Corps, and IV Corps. Created by Bill Lewis, former executive director of the New Jersey Agent Orange Commission, 1991-1996. Reproduced with permission.

Present day dioxin

If H5N1 cases and deaths in southern Vietnam are due to the combination of influenza and TCDD from food and soil, what is causing the sudden spike in cases and number of deaths from human bird flu cases in Indonesia, a country that has had no exposure to Agent Orange?

As of June 2006, Indonesia had reported 50 human H5N1 infections and 38 deaths. Particularly disturbing was a cluster of cases that occurred in May involving eight family members, seven of whom died. All but one person in the family appeared to have caught the virus from another family member, making this the first known incidence of H5N1 spreading from one person to another, and then another. Alarmed officials feared that the bird flu virus had acquired characteristics that would soon allow easy passage from human-to-human.

The deceased family lived in a small village in Karo district located in the Indonesian province of North Sumatra. The Karo highland borders on Lake Toba, the world's largest volcanic lake and the largest lake in Southeast Asia. The lake has been deteriorating since 1998, defenseless against the onslaught of the province's pulp and paper mills.

The largest polluter of the lake for the past decade has been Indorayon, a paper, pulp and rayon manufacturer owned by multinational companies and funded by the World Bank. The mill was forced into temporary closure in 1998 by a grassroots revolt over the company's destruction of the local environment, but in 2003, yielding to pressures of its investors and international bankers, the government allowed the pulp portion of Indorayon to reopen under the name of PT Toba Pulp Lestari.

The company's pulp mills are still blamed for far-reaching environmental degradation due to the continued release of dangerous chemicals: chlorine and chlorine oxide, organochlorines, and dioxins, including TCDD. Furthermore, extensive deforestation throughout North Sumatra has had a devastating impact on local residents through mudslides, fluctuations in the water supply, and contamination of plants and fish.

An explosive number of pulp and paper mills have been built in Southeast Asia, Indonesia, and China over the last 15 years while local communities have protested the pollution caused by the mills with little success. Pulp mills are one of the most polluting industrial processes in the world. Much of that pollution is the result of the three million tons of chlorine used annually to bleach paper white. Chlorine bleaching is a major source of the potent carcinogen dioxin, which is routinely discharged into rivers and streams with wastewater.

As of 2005, there were seven pulp mills, 65 paper mills, and 10 pulp and paper mills in Indonesia. Is this the reason that bird flu outbreaks—resulting in human deaths—are occurring exponentially throughout Indonesia ?

The Phoenix pulp and paper mill in Thailand, a US$1 billion Chinese-Thai project, aims to double its capacity to 700,000 tons a year by using inexpensive loans from the Finnish and Swedish governments. The Taiwanese-Cambodian joint venture, Pheapimex, plans to build a US$70 million pulp and paper mill in Cambodia. In Laos, BGA Lao Plantation Forestry is planting 50,000 hectares of mainly eucalyptus plantations to feed a wood chip mill that will be exported to Japan. In Vietnam, Sweden's aid agency, Sida, with support from the Swedish Export Credit Corporation, is funding the expansion of the Bai Bang pulp and paper mill. Recently, the Vietnamese government announced plans for a new pulp mill project in Kontum province.

(Source: The Pulp Invasion: The International Pulp and Paper Industry in the Mekong Region, by Chris Lang. Published in WRM Bulletin 58, May 2002. http://chrislang.blogspot.com/2002 05 25 chris lang archive.html)

Contamination in China

China denied the presence of bird flu in humans throughout all of 2004. That changed, however, in December 30, 2005, when China reported to the WHO seven deaths scattered across six of its provinces: Anhui, Fujian, Guangxi, Hunan, Jiangxi, and Liaoning.

Agricultural authorities who were expeditiously dispatched to outbreak locations found a few dead ducks and chickens in the vicinity of the ill persons, blaming the birds for causing the outbreak. As with Vietnam and Thailand, there is more to the story.

All across this expansive country, there are millions of farmers living in close proximity to billions of chickens. Many virologists around the world have questioned the relative paucity of human cases in China, given that there have been at least 30 HPAI outbreaks among poultry scattered across ten different provinces since mid-October 2005.

While deaths may be going unreported, the conditions for increasing the number of bird flu cases are ripe. Strong economic growth, coupled with increased nationwide egg production, has led to a huge increase in egg consumption by the Chinese. The world's second largest per capita egg consumer (after Japan), China is consuming 292 eggs per person on a yearly basis. This represents nearly one egg a day, or possibly as much as 45 ppt of dioxin per day just from eggs alone.[16] While China's eggs were not part of the international dioxin and POP egg analysis, the poor environmental conditions throughout the country reflect the toxic exposures of the country's inhabitants. Throughout history, China's people have depended on the waters supplied by her seven major rivers for life itself. But over the last 20 years, water quality has deteriorated to a grave state.

The Yellow River, long regarded by the Chinese as the birthplace of their civilization, has been so heavily overused for consumption, irrigation, and factory production that the amount of water flowing through this once powerful river is occasionally reduced to nothing more than a trickle. According to the 2001 World Bank report, *China: Air, Land, and Water—Environmental Priorities for a New Millennium,* 40 percent of the water in large stretches of the Yellow River has been classified as "unsuitable for human contact, irrigation, and agriculture."[17] The list of river pollutants, both lengthy and disgusting, includes industrial chemicals, heavy metals, dead animals, and untreated human excrement. Couple this with nuclear waste that starts at the river's headwater in Tibet, it is only a matter of time before millions of Chinese become chronically ill.

The Chinese State Environment Protection Administration reports that industrial animal farms have become a major source of pollution. In 1995, for example, more than 1.7 billion metric tons of unprocessed manure was dumped into rivers that serve as water supplies.[18]

For China's second largest river, the Yangtze, conditions are much the same. More than 23.4 billion tons of sewage and industrial waste are dumped into the Yangtze each year and 15 percent of water samples taken in 2001 were classified as "unsuitable for human contact." That percentage, is certainly greater since 2001, and will continue to increase with the westernization of the Chinese culture.

The influx of rural peasants into cities has stretched the sewage infrastructure beyond all reasonable capacity. Deceptively, the operators of most new buildings report that the structures are connected to sewers, but none of the waste is being treated; up to 80 percent of raw sewage is still released directly into the water supply.[19]

In Northeast China, the Liao He is the principal waterway flowing to the Yellow Sea from Shenyang, the capital of Liaoning Province. In 1999, this river was classified as "only suitable for industrial purposes that do not involve direct human contact with the water."[20] Surely, it is far more contaminated by 2006. It should be no surprise that Liaoning Province has been the location of three out of the seven reported human cases of avian flu and many large outbreaks among poultry.

Beyond the severe problems of contaminated water, China is home to nine of the ten cities with the world's worst air pollution. Respiratory diseases linked to air pollution are the leading cause of death among both children and adults throughout China, according to a November 1999 report by the World Resources Institute, *Urban Air Pollution Risks to Children: A Global Environmental Health Indicator.* Chronic obstructive pulmonary disease (COPD) and pneumonia are the leading contributors of death in adults and children, respectively.[21]

Air pollution causes millions of Chinese to suffer from health ailments including lung cancer and decreased immune function. The air is so bad throughout southern China that in Yunnan Province women were found to be among those with the highest rates of lung cancer ever recorded: 125.6 cases per 100,000 women, compared to U.S. national averages of 6.3 per 100,000.[22]

The symptoms and diagnoses of the seven Chinese patients who were hospitalized (late 2005) and then confirmed with H5N1 have been catalogued in great detail by the WHO. All seven cases developed symptoms of fever, cough, respiratory distress, and pneumonia; two were children. Conditions for developing pneumonia, can include inhaling fumes and other toxic airborne particles. To expel the congestion, an overabundance of mucous is produced, creating the perfect environment for the rapid replication of the invading organisms. If the mucous contains a mixture of dioxin and other chemicals, the likelihood of death from influenza could be exponential.

Other than their conditions at the time of death, nothing else is known about the health of these patients. Considering that COPD and pneumonia are among the most common causes of death in China, the identification of H5N1 may have had little to do with their demise. Perhaps the cause of their pneumonia was environmental toxicities *complicated by the presence of H5N1*. Because tests are not performed to confirm the presence of heavy metals or environmental chemicals in these patients, the true cause of death among these patients will always be an uncertainty.

More outbreaks: Turkey

The media is obsessed with reporting every new "outbreak" of H5N1 discovered anywhere in the world. They are making good use of Rule No. 2 in the New Playbook, "Don't be afraid to frighten people" because "we can't scare people enough," as discussed in chapter six. In addition, continuing to report "new cases" justifies the ongoing expenditures for massive culling, vaccine development, Tamiflu stockpiling, regulation implementation, and international meetings. An example of blow-by-blow reporting occurred over a small cluster of outbreaks that occurred in mountainous eastern regions of Turkey in January 2006.

Located in the far northeastern corner of the country, Dogubayazit is approximately 35 miles from the Armenian border.

It was in this city of 50,000 inhabitants that three children were the first reported bird flu deaths in the country. Doctors blamed the outbreak on exposure to sick chickens while officials blamed the appearance of H5N1 on migratory birds. In the city of Van, 75 miles away, 15 people suspected of having bird flu were treated at Van University Hospital. Although no cases were confirmed, the reports of "an outbreak of bird flu" were boomed across hundreds of news outlets worldwide.

As in all other locations where the virus has been detected, poor people have been forced to hand over their healthy turkeys and chickens, watching in desperation as authorities stuffed them into sacks where they would suffocate while being buried alive. By January 8, 2006, 11 cities throughout Turkey had been quarantined, and the government had ordered the destruction of more than 4,000 chickens throughout six large eastern provinces.[23]

Van City, with a population of more than 300,000, is one of the most urbanized, industrialized, and agriculturally developed areas of east Turkey. The city is located on the eastern shore of Van Lake, the largest lake in Turkey and the fourth largest lake in the world. Van Lake has no outlet; it receives its water from numerous streams and rivers from the north and the east.[24] Because of the lake's high salinity, most of the municipality's water for its many inhabitants is supplied from groundwater wells. Fresh water is derived directly from the extensive underground supply, called an aquifer, which unfortunately can become contaminated by harmful surface chemicals and pose significant risks to humans. Since environmental pollution does not respect man-made boundaries, chemicals can adversely affect the air and water supply hundreds of miles from their source.

Turkey's neighbor, Armenia, is geographically part of the Caucasus region, the oldest connecting route between Europe and Asia. Formed after the breakup of the U.S.S.R. in 1991, Armenia, Georgia, and Azerbaijan are now independent countries in the southern Caucasus; the North Caucasus remains a part of the Russian Federation. Surprisingly, much information is available about the environmental conditions that existed throughout the Caucasus states when still part of the former Soviet Union. The heavy chemical and industrial contamination that occurred for many years throughout the region is no doubt affecting the inhabitants, the land, and the underground water supply of neighboring Turkey.

Poor water quality has long been a concern throughout the Caucasus region. Similar to the great rivers of China, the rivers and lakes throughout Armenia and Turkey are heavily contaminated from years of neglect and industrial abuse. Beginning in the Soviet era, large volumes of chemicals have been discharged from industrial and agricultural sources, causing pollution of both surface and ground waters. For example, the highly-polluted Aras (Araks) River, a major tributary of the Kura River that forms the boundary between Turkey and Armenia, courses across several countries before emptying into the Caspian Sea. The water is loaded with solid debris and choked by high sediment loads resulting from excessive deforestation. Agricultural run-off of pesticides and herbicides has caused oxygen-choking algae blooms to occur, killing off fish and other species of water wildlife. Polluted rivers carry industrial contaminants—ammonia, arsenic, heavy metals, oil products, phenols, and other hazardous substances—to cities and communities far downstream. Surface water can also contaminate the underground aquifer.

Population growth and urbanization throughout the southern Caucasus states and eastern Turkey have resulted in a many-ton increase of municipal wastes. Historically, solid waste was taken to landfills, covered with dirt, or burned. Since 1990, landfills in Armenia have been constantly overloaded, improperly operated, and are below minimum health and environmental requirements. Since the dumpsites leak chemicals, the soil and the underground water supply are poisoned. Open-pit mining operations spew massive amounts of chemicals openly into rivers and lakes, and there have been reports of large quantities of obsolete and banned pesticides, stored for more than 15 years in outdated, unsecured regional warehouses, contributing to massive contamination.[25]

In addition to chemicals, regional rivers are highly contaminated with human sewage. From the headwaters to the sea, very few treatment facilities exist. In the large municipalities, the plants are not capable of processing the amount of refuse they receive; in small villages, the untreated sewage is released directly into the river. Countless tons of untreated sewage is discharged into the Kura-Araks Rivers each year, with contamination levels exceeding international standards by 10 to 100 times.[26] During the annual spring melt, mountain runoff swells the rivers beyond their banks, spreading toxic contents across agricultural lands and villages where contamination enters the food chain for free-ranging chickens, migratory birds, and humans.

In addition to the hundreds of tons of toxic compounds and human sewage defiling the land and water, the region is choked by radioactive waste released by the nuclear power plant located in Metzamore, Armenia, a short 10 miles from the Turkish border where the H5N1 outbreaks were first reported in early 2006. The lack of natural energy resources led land-locked Armenia to approve building two reactors, referred to as the Armenian Nuclear Power Plant (ANPP) in 1976 and 1979, despite the fact that Armenia is located in a seismically active region. Strong pressure from an international coalition resulted in the plant closing down in 1988. During the years when the ANPP was inactive, electricity was available throughout the country for only one or two hours a day. The impact of electrical shortages was immeasurable in human and economic terms. Therefore, despite its location in an earthquake-prone zone and despite outrage by environmental groups, Armenia had few other options but to reopen the ANPP in 1995.[27] The *Caucasus Environmental Outlook Report of 2002* expressed concern that practically no data exists on nuclear waste handling or disposal during the 12 years between the plant's construction in 1976 and its temporary closing in 1988. When the plant was closed, the risk of groundwater contamination increased substantially for humans and animals alike.

In October 2005, the ANPP was shut down for a six-week maintenance program. On November 17, Armenia's general director, Gagik Markosyan, said the plant's sole working reactor was started up after being refueled with US$14.5 million in nuclear fuel supplied by Russia.[28] Perhaps it was not coincidental that just two months later, the Turkish Health Ministry began to confirm sick chicks and human deaths from H5N1 in Dogubayazit near the

Armenian border: It is unknown if nuclear waste or nuclear radiation had been accidentally released during the refueling process.

Spreading toward Europe: Ankara and beyond

Bird flu news warns that the virus is spreading across Turkey and "heading for Europe." Most likely, "outbreaks" *will occur* in other parts of Europe, and other parts of the world, but not for the reasons being expounded by the news. Chemical manufacturing plants are located in nearly every emerging country around the globe, and contamination from these facilities knows no boundaries. Coupling chemical contamination with the need for Tyson-like companies to expand their market share, Turkey and Eastern Europe are no doubt examples of things to come.

The chemical industry in Turkey is composed of more than 6,000 production facilities for petrochemicals, fertilizers, paints, pharmaceuticals, soaps and detergents, cosmetics, synthetic resins, and plasticizers. With nearly 2,500 products, the Turkish chemical manufacturing sector is robust.[29] As of April 2001, Turkey boasted more than 186 foreign investors in its chemical sector, including Dow Chemical, Bayer, Hoechst, Sandoz, Roche, GlaxoWelcome, BASF, Pfizer, and DuPont, generating at least US$14 billion in annual revenues with projected growth of 4 percent annually. The manufacturing facilities, scattered across the western part of the country, are mostly located in Istanbul, Izmir, Kocaeli, Adana, and Ankara. With little or no attention to the proper disposal of chemical waste, it is only a matter of time before more sick chickens, sick migratory birds, and sick humans are identified.[30]

In March 2005, the International POPs Elimination Network (IPEN) conducted an analysis of dioxin and other chemicals from the eggs of free-range chickens in Kosice City, the second largest city in eastern Slovakia. Composite samples of eggs from Kokshov-Baksha and Valaliky, "suburbs" of Kosice City, exceeded 10 times the background levels for dioxin in eggs established by the WHO.[31] With concentrations similar to those found throughout Southeast Asia, consumption of dioxin-laden eggs, increases the likelihood of significant problems in humans.

It should be no surprise that sick birds have been reported in various countries in Eastern Europe. Beyond the horrible ongoing pollution from incinerators and the booming chemical industry in the region are the remains of another war–from NATO air strikes– and the War in Kosovo beginning on March 24, 1999.

Excerpts from Dr. Janet Eaton's testimony at the International Tribunal for the U.S./NATO War Crimes in Yugoslavia mention the research of Dr. Radoje Lausevic of the University of Belgrade and the Serbian Ecological Society. He recorded the following list of chemicals that were released into the atmosphere, water, and soil during the NATO bombing of the Balkan states: oils and petroleum products, polychlorinated biphenyls (PCBs) ammonia, ethylene dichloride, sodium hydroxide, hydrogen chloride (1,000 tons released into rivers), vinyl chloride monomer (VCM) (1,000 tons released), phosgene, nitrogen oxides, hydrofluoric acid, heavy metals, carbon monoxide, aldehydes, soot, and particulates. Black clouds containing petrochemicals, mercury, and other pollutants from burning oil refineries and fertilizer plants delivered contaminates across a 20,000 square mile area. These continue to exist today.[32]

The chemical contamination accumulated from past–and present– wars may be contributing to the immunosuppression and the increased susceptibility of local residents to the inflammatory effects of H5N1.

Another issue of radiation: DU in Iraq

Since 1991, Iraq has been subjected to pollution through the use of using depleted uranium weapons launched by the U.S. and its Allies during Gulf War I. Depleted uranium, known as DU, is the by-product of the process that separates natural uranium from fissionable uranium used in nuclear bombs and for reactor fuel. Accumulating in the soil essentially forever, DU remains radioactive for about 4.5 billion years. When missiles containing DU hit the ground, they ignite on impact, releasing a firestorm of DU oxide particles into the air. The extremely fine residue of uranium dust can be carried by the wind, contributing to the absorption of the poison by humans, plants, and animals in distant locations miles away.[33]

The U.S. Army acknowledges the hazards of DU in its training manual. It requires anyone who comes within 75 feet (25 meters) of DU-contaminated equipment to wear respiratory and skin protection, stating that "contamination will make food and water unsafe for consumption." One outspoken activist, Dr. Doug Rokke, an Army health physicist assigned in 1991 to the command staff of the Twelfth Preventive Medicine Command and Third U.S. Army Medical Command headquarters, is speaking out about the human consequences of DU in Iraq. Called back into active duty from his research job in the Physics Department at the University of Illinois, Rokke was sent to the Gulf, along with a team of 100 professionals, to take charge of the DU cleanup operation. As it turns out, Rokke and his entire team performed their tasks without any specialized training from the Army and without protective gear. Today, at least 30 members of his team have died from the consequences of extreme radiation exposure, and most of the others, including Rokke, have serious health problems.

Attesting to the health consequences of the DU exposure, Rokke commented, "Verified adverse health effects from personal experience, physicians, and from personal reports from individuals with known DU exposures include reactive airway disease, neurological abnormalities, kidney stones and chronic kidney pain, rashes, vision degradation and night vision losses, lymphoma, various forms of skin and organ cancer, neuropsychological disorders, uranium in semen, sexual dysfunction, and birth defects in offspring. This whole thing is a crime against God and humanity."[34]

A major study completed in 2001 by three leading international radiation scientists cautioned that humans could contract cancer after exposure to DU dust. The paper was blocked from publication by the WHO. The lead researcher on the study, Dr. Keith Baverstock, WHO's top expert on radiation and health for 11 years, revealed after his retirement in 2003 that he was refused permission to publish the study.

217

"I believe our study was censored and suppressed by the WHO because they didn't like [our] conclusions. Previous experience suggests that WHO officials were bowing to pressure from the International Atomic Energy Agency (IAEA), whose [role] is to promote nuclear power," he said. "That is more than unfortunate, as publishing the study would have helped forewarn the authorities of the risks of using DU weapons in Iraq."

Baverstock's study suggested that the low-level radiation from DU could harm cells adjacent to those that are directly irradiated, a phenomenon known as "the bystander effect." This undermines the strength of the body's immune system, leading to the development of cancers and other illnesses. Baverstock went on to point out that the DU used in Iraq could have been contaminated with plutonium and other radioactive waste, making it more radioactive and hence more dangerous.[35]

Is it any wonder that bird flu cases are now being identified in Iraq?[36]

Putting it all together, the accumulation of dioxins, POPs, nuclear wastes and environmental pollutants is reaching a critical tipping point on the planet. The correlation between chemical toxicity and the circumstances in which H5N1 can proliferate have not been examined by health professionals or WHO officials. This failure is most likely due to their myopic fixation with the germ theory of disease. Identifying conditions in which a pandemic could emerge would be markedly more constructive.

*Reality is that which, when you stop believing
in it, doesn't go away.*
~Philip K. Dick, Writer/Filmmaker

Chapter 17: Tying It All Together

Starting points:
- The health of the terrain
- Why avian flu could happen here…but not for the reasons cited in the media
- Environmental wake-up call: What needs to be done

W hat do sick chicks, sick people in Southeast Asia, and sick migratory birds all have in common? An unhealthy immune system better described as an unhealthy terrain.

The health of the terrain

We have all been taught that germs are bad and that they are everywhere, lurking around every corner, waiting for the opportunity to invade defenseless humans. We go to great lengths to combat these potential invaders; we employ frequent hand-washing with copious amounts of soap and grimace at the thought of eating a morsel of food picked up from the floor. Doctors and the media discuss the flu season as though "getting the flu" is inevitable without the flu shot. But similar to other concepts in modern medicine that have been unquestioningly accepted, perceived human frailty is a medical myth. A better understanding of the relationship of the immune system between humans and microbes is necessary to

219

achieve optimal health.

The immune system is the name given to the complex interaction between white blood cells, antibodies, hormones, enzymes, and inflammatory molecules called cytokines, which act in synchrony to maintain health. Every moment, the body is exposed to billions of microbes living on the skin, in the mouth, in the digestive tract, and on everything we touch. Microbes that coexist with humans and animals are called symbiants—organisms that have developed a mutually beneficial relationship with the body and are considered to be part of the body's normal flora. The immune system recognizes organisms that don't belong in the body and effectively eliminates them. This process occurs thousands of times per day with little or no fanfare. However, it is not the invasion by external microbes that leads to symptoms known as an infection; it is the compromise of the immune system due to contamination of the terrain.

One of the basic differences between conventional medical practitioners and those who embrace alternative, or integrative, medical practices is their different interpretations of the impact that the Germ Theory of Disease (credited to Louis Pasteur) has had on healthcare. A discussion of its validity generally elicits divisiveness and even hostility among medical doctors and laypersons alike because the germ theory is the cornerstone of a large portion of modern medicine. Pasteur's mechanistic idea of disease—finding the right cure (drug) for each germ—engendered the growth of the pharmaceutical empire and its dominance over medicine today. It is most unfortunate that his premise was accepted to the exclusion of all others.

Pasteur is considered one of the luminaries of science. Some of his discoveries were undoubtedly noteworthy. For example, his discovery of the existance of microbes set the groundwork for minimizing the spread of disease in hospitals, and his work with rabies was the beginning of the study of viruses. Perhaps most famously, he has also been credited with the development of pasteurization, a method by which microbes are destroyed by heat without supposedly causing harm to food.

Rewriting generally accepted history is a monumentally

difficult task, especially when it involves a critical assessment of someone with the stature of Pasteur. However, there is another view of disease that challenges Pasteur's 150-year-old premise: Health is about the condition of the body called the "terrain," or the "soil." Only when the terrain is disrupted and contaminated will pathogens have an opportunity to propagate.

The germ theory and the opposing view about the body's terrain are part of the fabric of the history of medicine. Many notable individuals throughout the late 1800s and early 1900s were involved with the debate, but the most vocal and visible figures were Pasteur and his two contemporaries, Claude Bernard and Antoine de Béchamp, both strong critics of Pasteur's work. Bernard, a physiologist considered to be the father of experimental medicine, declared to a group of physicians and scientists, "The terrain is everything; the germ is nothing." His bold statement created the debate that has continued to this day.

What is little known about the germ theory, however, is that throughout his career, Pasteur had doubts about his own assumptions. Pasteur and Bernard frequently debated whether germs produced disease or whether the body's resistance was more important. Pasteur placed more emphasis on the microbe, while Bernard focused more on the environment, the terrain, in which the microbe could exist. On his deathbed, Pasteur said, *"Bernard avait raison. Le germe n'est rien, c'est le terrain qui est tout."* ("Bernard was right. The germ is nothing; the soil is everything.")[1] The germ theory of disease had become so profitable, however, even in Pasteur's day, that modern medicine dismissed his final confessions as nothing more than the ramblings of a dying man.

It bears repeating: The money is in the *medicine*—not the *cure*.

Bernard's view was that disease is an "inside-out job," meaning that when the physiology of the body becomes disrupted by pollutants common to industrialized societies—vaccines, chemicals, pesticides, heavy metals, processed food, preservatives, etc.—an environment is created for microbes to "set up shop" through the shifting of the acid-base balance of the body (pH) toward an acidic state. Acidity decreases a cell's ability to properly utilize oxygen. Without that vital process, enzymes malfunction and the body accumulates intracellular wastes instead of eliminating them. For the medically minded, acidic pH shifts compromise the energy production of the Krebs cycle and disrupts the efficiency of cytochrome p450 in the liver, the complex enzyme system that eliminates drugs from the body. When these systems start to break down, according to Bernard, cells begin to die, marking the beginning of disease.

Support for this concept comes from *Guyton's Textbook of Medical Physiology,* which teaches that one of the foundations for maintaining health is to normalize the pH, or balance the acid/alkaline ratio. When cells become acidic, virtually all functions in the body are affected.

Once compromise occurs, pathogens can find a favorable environment in which to replicate. As contrary as it seems, germs are attracted to the diseased tissues; they are not the primary cause of it. A quote from Dr. Rudolph Virchow, the father of modern pathology, supports this idea: "If I could live my life over again, I would devote it to proving that germs seek their natural habitat—diseased tissue— rather than being the cause of the diseased tissue; in other words, mosquitoes seek the stagnant water, but do not cause the pool to become stagnant."[2] The symptoms generally described as the flu, or identified as pneumonia—fever, chills, cough, and excess mucous production—are actually secondary illnesses. The first illness was loss of health in the underlying tissues and a broken immune system.

In fact, it may very well be that microbes, both bacteria and viruses, are here on the planet to induce the highly reactive inflammatory responses, modified cytokine storms, helping the body detoxify. It would be very illuminating to test the secretions that are expelled during a bout of the flu for chemicals and heavy metals. Instead of being the problem, viruses may be part of the solution, acting as the "clean-up crew," assisting the body to detoxify and eliminate the remains of chemicals, pharmaceutical drugs, heavy metals including mercury, and other environmental insults. It should be emphasized that the human race evolved *because of* its relationship to microbes, *not in spite of it.*

For example, if a person reportedly died from "viral pneumonia," perhaps the body was trying to expel a huge amount of chemical-containing mucous. If the person was too weak to muster an adequate immune response, or his lymphatics were too congested to drain the accumulated debris–and more chemicals were added during the acute episode, such as aspirin, antibiotics, anti-inflammatories, and steroids–the person may have become overwhelmed, leading to his demise. The death was blamed on the virus, but the *real* cause of death may well have been the person's inability to survive the detoxification process.

In the toxic world we live in, could it be that microbes are handy to have around? Could the purpose of microbes be to inflame the system, purging and cleaning out the muck? The Germ Theory would have us believe that microbes are "out to get us." Perhaps a reassessment is in order. Perhaps humans and germs should learn how to work together. Instead of fearing an episode of "the flu"–with its increased mucous, cough, fever, and diarrhea–we should view it as an act of cleaning out the internal dross. (After all, if our terrain were healthy, our detoxification processes fully functional, and our immune system intact, we would not "catch" the flu.

Instead of curbing the fever and stifling the cough with Western medicine's suppressive tools, supporting the elimination process with copious pure water, Vitamin C, homeopathy, herbs, and Chinese medicine is a much better way to regain health. In the long run, working *with* this elimination process may ultimately be the key to individual and species survival. Obviously, this novel concept would require a monumental paradigm shift to become widely accepted and would be met with great resistance. But for each individual, it is certainly worthy of consideration.

One of the systems of medicine that supports the belief that the person's ability to get well comes from within is osteopathic medicine. The teachings of osteopathy are parallel with, but separate from, conventional medicine.

Little known by most, osteopathic medicine was founded by a medical doctor, Andrew Taylor Still, who received his medical degree from the College of Physicians and Surgeons in Kansas City, Kansas. Early in his career, he served as a state legislator and attained the rank of major during the Civil War. After the war, Still became increasingly disenchanted with the accepted medical practices of the early nineteenth century, which included bloodletting, blistering, and the administration of massive doses of mercury, antimony, arsenic, and other poisonous mineral purgatives thought to act as "tonics." These therapeutic regimens certainly killed large numbers who were unfortunate enough to undergo treatment at the hands of their doctors. Instead of poisoning the body with toxic substances, Still believed that the primary role of the physician was to facilitate the body's inherent ability to heal itself.

Although his intent was to improve the current system of medicine, not to create a new one, Still's ideas were completely rejected by his peers. The American Medical Association (AMA), founded in 1847, had little tolerance for therapies that did not use drugs and other chemical compounds to treat patients. In fact, the aims of the organization as set forth in its first charter were threefold: (1) the establishment of medical licensing laws that restricted the number of physicians in a given state, resulting in a more "stable economic climate" by inhibiting competition; (2) the destruction of existing medical schools, replacing them with fewer, non-profit institutions of learning that would provide training to a "smaller and more select student body"; and (3) the elimination of "heterodox medical sects" as unwelcome and competitive forces within the profession.[3] In other words, the AMA was formed to eliminate all other medical philosophies and systems in this country such as homeopathy, Chinese medicine, and herbology. Little has changed to the present day.

Determined that his theories of health and healing were in the best interest of patients and armed with a profound knowledge of human anatomy and physiology, Still established a new medical school in 1874, Kirksville College of Osteopathic Medicine, in Kirksville, Missouri. Osteopathic medicine was developed to facilitate natural healing processes by finding and correcting structural abnormalities that could interfere with the free flow of blood and lymph fluid. Simple, manual techniques, such as lymphatic drainage, were taught to patients that helped to normalize the flow of fluids, eliminate toxicities, and restore health to the individual.[4] The principles of osteopathy—assisting the immune system to function fully and helping the body to heal itself—persist, but are used far less than they should be. This type of healthcare should be mainstream medicine, not "alternative medicine."

Unfortunately, investigating methods to restore health are rarely on the minds of researchers. For example, the large numbers of persons who have been exposed to H5N1 and have not gotten sick or have fully recovered from an illness presumed to be caused by the virus have received little attention. In our fear-based, drug-driven society, emphasis is placed on the death rate, not on the survival rate.

That small change in emphasis alters the entire structure of the discussion. For example, during the smallpox commotion, the death rate was continually publicized at a frightening 30 percent. Never was the 70 percent survival rate mentioned. The same can be said for the harping about bird flu.

If 30 children are in a classroom and five become ill with strep throat or a cold, what is it about the innate health of the other 25 that enabled them to remain well? Should we not be studying the healthy? Discovering the immune system properties that distinguish those who remain healthy in the presence of outbreaks, and finding ways to duplicate those properties in others, would be true science.

Bird flu: A wake-up call to global chemical contamination

Reports of H5N1 outbreaks are occurring throughout the world, and governments in Western Europe are now declaring the arrival of bird flu in their countries as "inevitable."[5] Perhaps they are right, but not for the reasons that are being reported.

Every day the environment becomes more contaminated with toxic industrial chemicals. Approximately 70,000 industrial chemicals have been registered with the EPA for commercial use, and each year approximately 1,500 new chemicals are introduced into the marketplace. Over the last 50 years, humans have been exposed to at least *one million tons* of 3,000 different chemicals annually. That's 2 *billion* pounds of chemicals every year. When chemicals absorb into the body fat of humans, animals, and birds, they put them at risk of serious health problems. Incredibly, little is known regarding the risks of most chemicals to human health, as the vast majority have not been tested. In addition, the minimal testing that has been done has evaluated only the risk of being exposed to one chemical at a time—a test model that is completely irrelevant in our toxic world.[6]

The mission statement of the Environmental Protection Agency, taken directly from its website, is "To protect human health and the environment. Since 1970, EPA has been working for a cleaner, healthier environment for the American people." Considering the chemically contaminated state of our world and the condition of our health, that statement is scandalous.

A recent study conducted by the WWF (formerly the World Wildlife Federation) demonstrates that critical levels of pervasive contamination are occurring worldwide. In spring 2005, the WWF collected blood specimens from 13 families for analysis. This study was unique in that the specimens were gathered from three generations (grandmother, mother, and child) of a family in each of 12 European Union countries: Belgium (two families), Denmark, Finland, France, Germany, Greece, Hungary, Italy, Latvia, Poland, Sweden, and Luxembourg.

Analyzing the blood for 107 different POPs, researchers found 73 hazardous chemicals in all generations, with some of the highest levels in children. Each person (grandmother, mother, and child) was found to be contaminated with a cocktail of at least 18 man-made chemicals, including PCBs and DDT, which have been banned for decades.

Since 2003, the WWF has analyzed blood samples from more than 350 people; in all cases, the people were found to be contaminated with a mixture of persistent, highly toxic, man-made chemicals.[7] Even in Western societies, no one is immune to the onslaught of two billion pounds of chemicals being added to the toxic burden of our planet each year.

The chemical load in the U.S. is no doubt less than what is being experienced throughout Southeast Asia, China, and Europe, but chemicals exist in all of us. In 2001, a scathing documentary on the chemical industry, *Trade Secrets: A Moyers Report*, started with the death of Dan Ross, a 46-year-old man who died of a rare type of brain cancer. Convinced that his 23 years working with vinyl chloride had been the source of his illness, he and his wife had sued the companies who made the chemical, charging them with conspiracy. During the legal discovery process, hundreds of thousands of documents were uncovered that led journalist Bill Moyers through a shocking tale of cover-up and intrigue. Confidential papers revealed a campaign to limit the regulation of toxic chemicals, eliminate any liability for their effects, and withhold vital information about risks from workers, the government, and the public.[8]

As part of his investigation into *Trade Secrets*, Moyers had his own blood tested for a large number of chemicals through a pilot study sponsored by the Mount Sinai School of Medicine in New York City. Even though he had no history of exposure, 84 chemicals were detected in his blood and urine samples, including 13 dioxins and furans. The list of chemicals included 17 that were toxic to the immune system and 48 that were known carcinogens.[9] Because these highly specialized laboratory tests are expensive, routine testing is not carried out for the general public. The same battery of tests performed on Moyers would cost an individual more than $6,000.[10]

Another shocking study, completed in September 2004, revealed how dangerously pervasive chemicals in the environment have become. It has long been held that the placenta acts like a shield, protecting the fetus from environmental chemicals and pollutants. However, that belief was blown apart by a first-of-its-kind study involving the umbilical cord blood of 10 newborn infants. Two major laboratories tested the specimens for more than 400 chemicals at a cost of more than $10,000 per sample. Researchers detected 287 chemicals in the cord blood. A breakdown confirmed that 180 were known carcinogens, 217 were known to be harmful to the central nervous system, and 208 have been proven to cause birth defects or abnormal development in experimental animals. Of the total, 11 were dioxins.[11] Even when precious infants enter the world, their bodies contain a load of toxic chemicals.

The sum of all industrial chemicals, pollutants, and pesticides accumulated in the fat of humans, animals, and birds over time is referred to as the "total body burden." Besides chemicals, other substances that contribute to the toxic load include heavy metals (mercury, cadmium, antimony, lead, etc.), food additives (such as MSG and aspartame), and prescription medications (such as antibiotics and vaccines). Although each compound has its own significant impact, the most important contaminant contributing to this discussion regarding bird flu is dioxin.

As of January 2006, the largest number of bird flu-related deaths have been in Vietnam. Because little is known about the persons who reportedly died from H5N1 in Cambodia, and Thailand, perhaps those persons were originally from or had spent significant time in Vietnam. To illustrate: 2,279 Vietnamese immigrants were granted Thai nationality in the largest naturalization in the country's history on January 3, 2006. It will remain unknown if those who died in Southeast Asia had a history of living in Vietnam and had experienced high levels of dioxin exposure, as the migration patterns in that part of the world are not documented.[12]

It is highly unlikely that the bird flu in humans is he result of farmers living in close proximity to their chickens. Consider the paucity of infections in other Third World countries where humans have lived in close proximity to high-density poultry populations for decades.

For example, Bangladesh, with dismally poor hygienic conditions, is among the poorest populations in the world. There, an estimated 144 million people are compressed into a mere 55,600 square miles (144,000 square kilometers), an area slightly smaller than the state of Georgia. In recent years, the poultry industry has grown exponentially in Bangladesh. In 2005, the country was reported to have approximately 150,000 poultry farms with annual revenues of more than US$750 million. Although the industry

The principal dioxin-induced biologic responses occurring in both humans and experimental animal models include the following:

- Chloracne
- Cancer
- Endometriosis
- Altered sex hormone levels
- Altered developmental outcomes
- Altered thyroid function
- Altered immune function
- Altered cellular growth and differentiation
- Altered presence and functionality of the AhR gene

suffered substantial financial losses due to an HPAI outbreak in 2003, when 10,000 broiler farms and 50 "doc" (day old chicken) breeding hatcheries were closed down; no human cases were reported.[13] Likewise, throughout 2004 and 2005, Bangladesh reported no cases of H5N1 in poultry or in humans.[14] Similarly, even though there have been few **human cases** of bird flu in India, Burma (Myramar), Australia and Africa, and no cases in any other country in South America, it should come as no surprise when outbreaks in birds are reported more and more frequently, with the industry missing the mark on the cause.

For example, a poultry outbreak occurred in Nigeria, (February 2006) and migratory birds were immediately blamed.[15] Many experts figured the virus would spread rapidly among farms and into wild birds across the region; it did not. Neither did it spread to countries surrounding Nigeria or to Africa's other big lakes. Scientists stated that they just didn't understand the life cycle of the virus. More likely, they don't understand the underlying cause of the sick birds—chemical toxicity.

More than 50,000 tons of obsolete pesticides and seriously contaminated soils have accumulated throughout Africa over the last four decades. With less than 5 percent of the stockpiles being appropriately disposed of, creating a dangerous threat to the health of both rural and urban populations has been created. Due to the struggling economic situation across the continent, this toxic situation will continue to get worse: Removal of chemical stores is rarely perceived as a priority issue.[16]

Similar types of ecologic destruction caused by chemicals are occurring in South America. A recently opened pulp mill in Chile, and industry that releases massive amounts of dioxin, has devastated one of South America's most biologically outstanding wetlands, eliminating its famed population of black-necked swans along with most other bird life. "This was an area that was once teeming with water birds," said David Tecklin, World Wildlife Fund's eco-region coordinator. "Now, within the space of just months, it has become an empty expanse of brown, polluted water. It is a water desert. Words really can't describe the magnitude of the disaster here."[17]

When at least 47 migratory birds were found dead in northern

India, the investigation by the Indian Cranes and Wetlands Working Group said that the toxic chemical responsible for killing the birds may have been mercury. District authorities were also notified that highly toxic fertilizer had been used near the site of a bird sanctuary near Delhi, resulting in the daily deaths of dozens of crows and other birds.[18]

It is only a matter of time before "bird flu" arrives everywhere.

Consider this: "Garden variety," mildly pathogenic seasonal influenza infections and H5N1 infections have both been associated with mild symptoms, but garden variety virus coupled with dioxin can cause deadly disease. Because mortality from the flu will be limited to those who have a substantial total body burden of dioxin, it is unlikely that H5N1 will become a "pandemic" in the immediate future. Unfortunately, without funds for routine testing, sporadic cases of death in the presence of HPAI will no doubt occur, and without enforcing cleanup programs for global natural resources—food, water, and air—world citizens will continue to accumulate pollutants in their fat tissues. The risk of a pandemic outbreak will increase, but not because a virus has "swapped surface antigens" or "jumped species." It will occur due to increased contamination of the human terrain with dioxins.

The WHO has defined the TDI for dioxin as 0.01 ppt per day. For a 150-pound (70kg) adult, that is 0.7 ppt per day. In the study completed by Schecter et al., all 16 samples of Vietnamese food were found to have greatly elevated levels of dioxin, ranging from 48 ppt in chicken to 343 ppt in the fat of free-ranging ducks. Schecter pointed out that TCDD made the largest contribution to total toxicity in these foods.[19]

In comparison, three separate government agencies in the U.S. have established recommendations for a "safe" daily dose of dioxin. As much as 98 percent of the dioxin in American diets comes from meat, fish, and dairy products. Consequently, when these foods are consumed, dioxins accumulate in fat tissue. The average daily intake of dioxin for Americans is approximately 0.154 ppt per day—negligible compared to the daily load consumed by the Vietnamese.[20] Over time, it has been estimated that an average adult in the U.S. has a total dioxin load of 36 to 58 ppt contained in his body fat. This clearly establishes that the risk of an H5N1 pandemic in the U.S. is negligible.

Similarly, the level of dioxin in foods throughout the U.K. and Europe is negligible compared with the levels in the food sampled from Vietnam. The U.K. standards limit one to three ppt for meat and chicken, four ppt for fish, and two to three ppt in eggs. The new dietary TDI for the U.K. and Europe that went into effect in November 2001 named the allowable level at 0.14 ppt per day for an adult.[21]

The bottom line of all this tinkering by the WHO, the EPA, and other international governmental organizations to determine "safe levels" of a known carcinogen is absolute nonsense. A chemical that has been proven to cause cancer, neuro-developmental defects, reproductive toxicity, and increases the risk of death from influenza does not belong in the body. Regardless of scientific calculations and epidemiological surveys, there is *no safe dose of dioxin.* As with radiation, dioxin is dangerous at *any* level, no matter how small.[22]

Massive doses, many times the level of "safe dioxins," are being ingested by world citizens on a daily basis. Culling chickens and creating dangerous vaccines is not the answer. Stockpiling worthless drugs is not the answer. Cleaning up the environment, improving practices of animal husbandry, and eliminating corporate greed are the places to start.

Beyond Vietnam, the chemical contamination of developing countries is exploding out of control. In China, widespread use of fertilizers and pesticides have adversely affected rivers and the groundwater everywhere in that expansive country. The area around the heavily industrialized city of Shenyang in Liaoning Province, where the largest number of outbreaks of HPAI in poultry have occurred to date, is a vivid example. There, an irrigation canal built in the early 1960s that drains an average 100,000,000 gallons (400,000 m3) of untreated wastewater each day from coal mines and plants, include contaminants from petrochemical, power, and chemical facilities. These toxins are contributing to the poor health of local inhabitants. Between 1973 and 1984, a government survey determined that residents near the canal had approximately three times as many cases of liver cancer and approximately three times more birth defects than residents of control areas.[23] Even though it has been five years since China signed the Stockholm Convention on Persistent Organic Pollutants, mechanisms for measuring and controlling POPs in the environment have not been implemented. The environmental contamination is no doubt causing severe toxicity in domestic and migratory birds and in humans.

Heavy industrialization certainly plays a role in increasing a local population's exposure to levels of dioxin. For example, even though parts of Laos were sprayed by Agent Orange during the war, most subjects tested by the Laos Ministry of Health showed only low levels of dioxin. The researchers concluded that these levels were consistent with what would be expected in a primarily rural country with less industrialization and less industrial pollution."[24] In other locations, however, a combination of chemicals from war and chemicals from unenforced environmental policies is creating the perfect environment for bird flu.

Persistent organic pollutants and dioxins possess toxic properties, resist degradation, and accumulate in the fat of animals, birds, and humans. The chemicals can be transported by migratory species across international boundaries and deposited far from their place of origination. When released, they can accumulate in a new ecosystem, making it difficult to identify the origin of the compound. For example, if a migratory bird feeds in a particular area and its eggs are laid in the vicinity of the feeding grounds, the chemical content in its eggs would reflect local sources. However, if the bird feeds in one area and then migrates to a distant place to lay its eggs, those eggs would not reflect the levels of local contamination. Again, the original source of the chemical would be unknown.[25]

Therefore, although egg studies are useful as a measure of local contamination, chemicals found in the eggs of migratory birds can serve as a disturbing measure of worldwide industrial filth.

Wild ducks and geese are highly peripatetic, moving from one water locale to another, eating small fish living in contaminated water and plants growing from contaminated soil. The reported outbreaks among migratory birds must become a wake-up call for the world's countries and international organizations to get serious about improving the environment. The birds are nature's way of sending an urgent message of impending disaster, similar to the message of dead canaries in the coal mines.

The use of bright yellow canaries were coal miners' life insurance policy because the metabolism of the canaries is highly sensitive to the effects of methane and carbon monoxide—odorless but deadly gases. The birds would chirp and sing throughout the day, but if the concentration of toxic gases increased to dangerous levels, the birds would suffocate and die. The silence was a signal to miners that an explosion was imminent; the sacrificed birds bought them time to rush out of the mine to avoid disaster.

The deaths of wild and domestic birds are serving as a similar warning—we are at the point of global disaster. Sick domestic chickens are warning us that our local environment and the genetic manipulation of our food are reaching the tipping point. The mass culling of our early-warning messengers is akin to shutting off a blaring fire alarm without looking for a fire.

More than 100 million domestic chickens, ducks, geese, and turkeys in at least nine countries have been destroyed since December 2003 when H5N1 first appeared. Culling flocks may limit the immediate presence of the virus, but it won't stop a new virus from reappearing unless the living conditions and the overall health of the birds are improved. "When you have an enormous number of birds in disgusting conditions, you're setting yourself up for some really horrible things," says Robert Sprinkle, a physician and associate professor of public policy at the University of Maryland School of Public Affairs.[26] By placing new chicks in a sick environment, the cycle is bound to occur all over again.

It bears repeating: The dreadful living conditions for the industrially-raised chickens, coupled with multiple vaccines and environmental toxicities, have suppressed the immune systems of all the birds involved, leading to the increased susceptibility of an influenza catastrophe within the flocks.

The H5N1 virus will continue to be identified in other parts of the world. Recall that the H5N1 antibody has been found in the blood of thousands of humans who were completely asymptomatic. Assuredly, asymptomatic birds can be carriers of the H5N1 virus, making its presence irrelevant. Is the isolation of H5N1 in a dead bird necessarily the cause of the bird's death? Of course not. Does the presence of H5N1 *in a country* suggest that *all* the humans in that country are at risk? Again, of course not.

Or consider this: Perhaps this viral strain isn't a "novel" strain after all. Science can't find what it's not looking for, and now that everyone is frantically looking for H5N1, they're finding it. Maybe it has been around for a long time. No one noticed—or no one cared—until now, when it could provide distinct economic and political advantages.

The strongest argument for concern over the presence of H5N1 is its potential for combining with dioxin in the lungs. This combination has proven to create a highly lethal situation for birds and humans alike. Dioxin is capable of producing a multitude of harmful effects. Because genetics play a role in health, humans will differ in their susceptibility to the effects of this chemical. Factors such as gender, age, total toxic load, and the capacity of certain liver enzymes to eliminate environmental chemicals will determine individual reactions to a particular level of dioxin.

Because all humans contain some level of dioxin in their bodies, more research is needed to understand the ramifications of low-level, lifetime exposures on health.[27] The critical dioxin concentration necessary for the occurrence of an explosive cytokine storm is unknown. Certainly, many variables to this combination must exist. In the presence of H5N1, a person can be asymptomatic or have only mild symptoms. Therefore, a "significant minimum level" of dioxin must be established to know who is truly at risk.

The significance of pathogens in the body can be better understood through the following analogy:

> During October 2003, dumpsters overflowed throughout Chicago when trash collectors went on strike. Up to 15,000 tons of garbage accumulated daily, and as the piles mounted, so did the health risk to the city's residents. Rats began to gather within 48 hours after garbage was left on the streets. Because a study 20 years earlier had estimated the rat population at more than seven million, almost the

same as the human population for the metropolitan area, concerns rose at the specter of rats once again taking over the area.

Although the elimination of the rats received the most attention, the solution to the stinky problem in the city was not to poison all the rats—it was to eliminate the garbage; the rat problem would eventually take care of itself. Similarly, during an episode of cough, mucous production, and fever, the administration of antibiotics is not the answer in the long run. The only way to recover health is by getting rid of the garbage.

The 1918 pandemic revisited

The cornerstone argument for pushing the global agenda of massive pandemic preparation is the supposed similarity between the H5N1 virus to the virus that caused the Spanish flu in 1918. However, little attention has been given to the similar correlation between the global contamination with dioxin and the massive use of chemical warfare from 1915 to 1917, just prior to the outbreak of the Great Influenza Pandemic.

The *Leavenworth Papers,* published by the Combat Studies Institute for the U.S. Army at Fort Leavenworth, Kansas, in 1984, is a collection of monographs regarding military history and strategy. One paper in particular, *Leavenworth Paper No. 10,* chronicles "the introduction of chemical agents in World War I, the U.S. Army's tentative preparations for gas warfare prior to and after American entry into the war, and the AEF (Air Expeditionary Force) experience with gas on the Western Front." The following information has been summarized from this lengthy paper:

During World War I, chemists on both sides investigated more than 3,000 chemical substances for potential use as weapons. Of those, only 30 agents were used in combat, and only about a dozen achieved the desired military results. Most armies grouped war gases according to their physiological effects on the human body. The most important and most widely used was mustard gas.

Strictly speaking, mustard gas (dichlorethylsulphide) is not a gas, but a liquid, which slowly vaporizes at normal ambient temperatures. It could be removed from dugouts, trenches, and equipment by the addition of chlorine or bleaching powder. Mustard gas was known to be toxic in concentrations that could not be detected by the sense of smell. Persons affected suffered no discomfort when they were exposed, as the symptoms of severe burning and blistering did not become evident until many hours later. Mustard gas penetrated all clothing and was remarkably persistent on the earth or on foliage, increasing its effectiveness.

From 1915 forward, agents were introduced that could be deployed using shells instead of canisters. With the use of heavier artillery, soldiers didn't have to rely on wind direction to deliver the gas onto enemy troops. Shells also offered an element of surprise not available with cloud attacks. Finally, gas shells proved to be more advantageous than high explosive rounds alone because shells did not have to score direct hits on a target to neutralize it.

The Germans were responsible for introducing dozens of noxious agents into the war theater. For example, in May 1916 they began to use shells filled with diphosgene, a strong lung irritant. Later that year, shells were filled with a mix of 75 percent phosgene and 25 percent diphosgene. By July 1917 they used three different mixtures of phosgene, diphosgene, and diphenylchlorosine, a chlorine gas and shells filled with a fine dust of arsenic. In field trials, arsenic powder proved extremely effective, as it penetrated the filters of all masks in use. But it was "Yellow Cross" (mustard gas) that gave the Germans the distinct advantage in chemical warfare. When mustard gas was coupled with explosives, it could be spread over wide areas and kept airborne for an extended period.

On April 6, 1917, when the U.S. declared war on Germany, no one in the nation seemed to have any practical knowledge concerning chemical warfare equipment or how the Germans were using the chemicals. The Army not only lacked defensive equipment for chemical warfare, it also had no concrete plans to develop or manufacture gas masks or any other type of defensive equipment.

Extremely toxic chemicals were used on troops on both sides of the war. A complete list, insofar as is known, of the gases used by the enemy, includes the following:

acrolein	diphenylchlorarsine
allylisothiocyanate	diphenylfluorarsine
arsenic trichloride	ethyldichlorarsine
arsine	formaldehyde
bromacetone	hydrocyanic acid
bromacetic ether	hydrosulphuric acid
bromethylmethylktone	iodacetic ether
Bromide of benzyl	iodacetone
Bromide of xylyl	methylchlorsulphonic acid
Bromide of toluyl	monochlormethylchloroformate
bromine	(palite)
carbon monoxide	nitrogen peroxide
carbonyl chloride (phosgene)	phenylcarbylamine chloride
chloracetone	phosphine
chlorine	phosphorus trichloride
chloropicrin	sulphur dioxide
cyanogensdichlorethylsulphide	sulphur trioxides
(mustard gas)	trichlormethylchloroformate
dichlormethylether	(diphosgene or superpalite)
dimethylsulphate	

The Medical Department of the United States in the World War, Volume XIV, Medical Aspects of Gas Warfare, Washington: Government Printing Office, 1926.

Even if gas masks had been available, the Army would have had no idea how to use them during combat. By the summer of 1917, U.S. troops began to arrive at French ports without minimal preparations to protect themselves, even though chemical warfare had become commonplace. On the eve of the American intervention, more than 12,000 troops were advanced to within 30 miles of the front, all without gas masks or training in chemical warfare.

It wasn't until January 1918 that the U.S. military established gas training camps. They consisted of a brief lecture and gas mask drills lasting one hour a day, five days a week, under the close supervision of British instructors. The training included putting the masks on and taking them off while sitting in a chamber filled with chlorine gas. Next, the troops entered a chamber filled with a tear agent for five to 10 minutes where they continued to practice masking and unmasking under duress. At peak times more than 2,000 men a day were put through this initiation. By the summer of 1918, all recruits were required to receive this standardized chemical warfare training.

Experimentation on troops in the name of training has been going on for centuries. For example, a minimum of three surprise gas attacks were included as part of the drills. To test the alertness of sentries and to correct such "carelessness as leaving their masks out of reach," attacks were often scheduled at night while the troops were asleep. Men on firing ranges were exposed to surprise gas attacks to become familiar with operating equipment while under attack and to overcome the difficulty of firing a weapon while masked. During night marches, men were subjected to gas attacks to "teach them how to overcome confusion." Other types of drills included officers ordering men to walk through clouds of gas from opened cylinders to instill confidence in their training and equipment.[28]

In the Army, the tight quarters during travel increased the exposure to viruses among troops. During the day, three men crammed themselves into every double seat on the trains. In the sleeping cars, one man slept in the upper bunk and two in the lower. The intense physical training and chemical exposure the men underwent in camps helped to weaken their resistance and make them more susceptible to the flu.

The cramped quarters experienced by the naval recruits were no better. On August 27, 1918, the first case of the flu occurred in Boston at the Navy's Commonwealth Pier. Within two weeks, 2,000 officers and men of the First Naval District had the flu. By the end of September, the flu had struck Navy bases as far away as Louisiana, Puget Sound, and San Francisco, and Army camps from Massachusetts to Georgia to Washington.

The flu received little attention in Europe. In the civilian populations of Europe, urban dwellings were crowded, dirty, and poorly ventilated, with little or no public health sanitation available. Many surely felt that lethal epidemics had been a common part of their lives for centuries, having experienced firsthand, or having heard about, deaths from infectious outbreaks of one kind or another for generations. Learning that another disease was sweeping the world had little effect on those who had already survived centuries of plague, cholera, yellow fever, and malaria.[29]

The epidemic seemed to crest in England in June 1918; at the same time, milder versions appeared in China and Japan. In Asia it was called the "three-day fever" or sometimes, "wrestler's fever," suggesting that, similar to H5N1 outbreaks, mild cases of the Spanish flu occurred and fatal cases had a contributing factor.[30]

There are many estimates of the number of deaths that occurred as a result of the 1918 pandemic. The U.S. death toll among the military was reported to be 650,000; the Russians, 450,000; the Italians, 375,000; and the British, 228,000—many of them were soldiers returning from the battlefield. It has been discovered from military documents that soldiers were dying in France as early as 1916 from the flu. The bluish-purple discoloration of the victim's lips and skin linked the deaths to the Spanish flu.[31]

An unusual feature of the Spanish flu was the age-mortality curve. Flu usually kills young children and the elderly, but the 1918 flu largely took males between 19 and 34 years of age. The disease's effect on military age men was so great that the American draft was suspended in October of 1918 due to the outbreaks. As the Allies engaged Germany in a series of final offensives, the flu was said to be a major player in the overall mortality rate, swinging the outcome of some battles.

Although the *Leavenworth Papers* do not specifically list Fort Riley as a gas training camp, a strong possibility exists that enlisted men could have participated in gas training exercises prior to arriving at Fort Riley—the location credited for the start of the Spanish flu. Soon after the outbreak began, chemical-laden military troops were transported to Europe and other parts of the world, carrying with them an influenza virus that may have gotten started by an interaction with toxicities in the lungs.

For the three years prior to the first outbreak at Fort Riley, Kansas, thousands of tons of explosives had sent millions of pounds of toxic liquids and poisonous gases into the air over the military theater in Europe. The suspended chemicals could have traversed the globe, contaminating civilians in diverse places, increasing their risk to a fatal outcome from influenza. Fueled by the primitive public health conditions of the time, and a predilection of that particular virus to react with chemicals, the global influenza pandemic was ignited.

This is not as outrageous as it may sound. Pollen has been discovered deep in the ice of Antarctica. Dust from China has been delivered to the U.S. through the air after massive wind storms. The smoke and particulates from the massive timber fires in Indonesia were measured in the air on the other side of the globe. Satellite instruments showed that sulfur dioxide released during the eruption of Mt. Pinatubo, Philippines, in 1991, circumvented the globe in only three weeks, and then slowly dispersed to cover much of the Earth in the following two years.[32] The idea of phosgene, mustard gas, chlorine gases, and the 30-odd other chemicals released into the environment during three years of daily explosions finding their way around the globe and causing health problems thousands of miles from their course is not as outrageous as it may initially seem.

The end of the war came swiftly; the Germans requested a ceasefire on October 3, 1918, and by November 11 an armistice had been signed. By December 1918, approximately 18 months after the epidemic began, the outbreaks stopped and history reported that the Spanish flu "mysteriously disappeared."

The massive use of chemicals during WWI could be responsible for the major spike in susceptibility to influenza worldwide. (Recall that influenza coupled with dioxin can lead to deadly results.) With war chemicals such as phosgene, chlorine gas, and mustard gas and pre-deployment vaccines in soldiers creating a toxic terrain prior to the exposure of a potent virus, it makes sense that many people could become victims of a massive cytokine storm.

A key symptom in many sufferers was cyanosis, a blue discoloration of the face caused by rapid accumulation of fluid in the lungs. For patients who developed the grotesque, lavender-gray hue over their face and ears, imminent death from suffocation was a near certainty. Historical records reported that people without symptoms could be "struck suddenly" and rendered "too feeble to walk" within hours, dying as soon as the next day.

Does that sound like a case of the flu?

Although the connections between environmental contamination, war chemicals, sick birds, sick people, and the current outbreak of H5N1 have not been conclusively proven, the statistical, circumstantial, and historical evidence is compelling, demanding rigorous and objective study. Only a moderate amount of research would be necessary to sort out whether the alarm displayed over a potential pandemic—with viruses anticipated to jump species and cause worldwide death and pandemonium—is justified, or if the panic is totally contrived.

But objectivity and reason are nearly impossible when asking officials to point a guilty finger at chemical contamination and dreadful animal husbandry, the real reasons that birds and people are sick. The verdict would turn global planning and vested careers upside down. Public health representatives would be humiliated for creating a solution—mass vaccination—without addressing the underlying cause of the illness. The reputations of esteemed scientists would be irreparably tarnished for blundering the fundamental issue. Politicians would suffer career-ending condemnation for pouring billions of tax dollars into the frantic development of drugs and vaccines instead of allocating critically needed funds to clean up the environment.

Sadly, it appears that world governments have chosen to push an agenda that invokes fear of H5N1 instead of investigating the associations between the environment and the bird flu virus, and then holding the global polluters—chemical companies, drug companies, agribusinesses, and promoters of war—accountable.

The truth brings with it a great measure of absolution, always.
~R.D. Laing, Scottish Psychiatrist

Chapter 18: Getting Involved: The Activist's Playbook

Starting points:
- Drugs, chemicals, and agriculture: Masterful connections
- Getting involved

Agribusiness has created GM seeds that require chemicals to grow. The claim that GM grains would be environmentally friendly, with less chemical use, is the exact opposite of what has occurred. A report from Dr. Charles Benbrook, director of the Northwest Science and Environmental Policy Center in Idaho, concluded that the 550 million acres of GM corn, soybeans, and cotton planted in the U.S. from 1996 through 2003 increased pesticide use (herbicides and insecticides) by about 50 million pounds.[1] Reports in the medical literature of illnesses associated with pesticides include adult and childhood cancers, numerous neurological disorders, autoimmune disorders, asthma, allergies, infertility, miscarriages, and child behavior disorders including learning disabilities, hyperactivity, and ADD (attention deficit disorders). Imagine the staggering number of drugs—and their associated costs—used to treat each of these disorders that are really environmentally-induced illnesses.

Pharmaceutical companies, chemical companies, and agribusinesses are not separate industries, but function more as "sister enterprises," working together for combined benefit, profit, and power. They are not competitors, but synergists, creating massive wealth through designing drugs as solutions for the health problems caused by their chemical and pesticide products.

The connection between the industry giants is masterful. Here's one example:

The drug company AstraZeneca was formed as a result of a merger between U.K.-based, Zeneca, a leading manufacturer of industrial chemicals and pesticides, and the Swedish drug giant, Astra. In the year preceding the merger (1997), Zeneca had sales of US$8.62 billion, 49 percent from the sale of pesticides and other industrial chemicals and an additional 49 percent from pharmaceutical sales, most of which were drugs for the treatment of cancer.[2]

One of Zeneca's pesticides, acetochlor, is thought to be a causal factor in breast cancer.[3] It is licensed for use in the U.S. through a co-registration between Zeneca and another chemical giant, Monsanto. In 1994, The Environmental Working Group reported that several herbicides in the triazine family—atrazine, simazine, and cyanazine—were shown in repeated studies involving female rats to cause breast cancer. An increased risk of breast cancer in women is also suspected.[4]

The primary manufacturer of atrazine and simazine is Syngenta, formed by the merger between drug giant Novartis and Zeneca's agrochemical division. Two drugs made by NovartisOncology, a division of Novartis, , are Femara™, for treating breast cancer, and Zometa™, for treating breast cancer that has spread to the bones.[5]

It was Zeneca that founded National Breast Cancer Awareness Month in 1985, when it was still owned by Imperial Chemical Industries. It is AstraZeneca that contributes to every leaflet, poster, and cute little pink ribbon used in the annual campaign to encourage thousands of well-meaning citizens to "Run for the Cure."

AstraZeneca also makes Tamoxifen™, prescribed to prevent recurrence of breast cancer. Tamoxifen is a known carcinogen; it increases the risk of two types of cancer that can develop in the uterus: endometrial cancer, which arises in the lining of the uterus, and uterine sarcoma, which arises in the muscular wall of the uterus. According to the NIH and The Cancer Information Network, women who take Tamoxifen have twice the chance of developing uterine cancer compared with women taking a placebo.[6]

One of the drugs used to treat endometrial cancer, adriamycin, is manufactured by Pharmacia, Inc., the previous owner of GM grain giant, Monsanto.[7] It was Monsanto that made Agent Orange.

It was Syngenta's genetically modified corn, Bt 176™, soon to be approved for human use, that presumably led to the death of cows in Germany. Considering the fact that there have been virtually no independent studies of the health effects of GM foods, humans should take a lesson from the animals. When geese returned to a farm field in Illinois during their annual migration, they selectively refused to eat rows of soybeans that had been planted with Monsanto's GM soya.[8] The *Washington Post* reported in 1999 that rodents refused to eat GM tomatoes. When the tomatoes were force-fed to the animals through a tube placed into their stomach, 17 percent died within two weeks.[9]

They obviously know something we should know.

What to do next

After coming this far in exposing the connections to the real causes of bird flu and international plans for global compliance with "pandemic preparedness," the obvious question becomes "What do we do about it?" For those new to this type of information, anger mixed with frustration and helplessness can no doubt result.

My suggestion is to get involved. Get more informed. Take any issue discussed in this book that grabs you—stopping mandatory vaccination, boycotting GM food products, advocating animal rights (especially the humane handling of poultry), supporting environmental cleanup projects, or stopping the use of chemical warfare. Pick one that speaks to your heart and give it your all. For every issue there are organizations out their working feverishly to oppose corporate greed and increase accountability. They need your support, your finances, and, most importantly, your time. You can continue to sit complacently on the sidelines, or you can choose to make a difference.

On a personal level, eliminate as much toxicity from your life as you possibly can. By improving your health overall, you will improve your immune system. Clean up your diet by minimizing—or better, eliminating—refined white sugar, white flour, food additives, and other toxic components that you eat. Get a good home water filtration system. There are many well-written books available on these topics. Pick one and get started; which one you choose is much less important than that you simply begin.

Select a form of healing for yourself and your family that is outside the Western paradigm of using chemicals called "drugs" for something called "medicine." Conventional treatments view illness as an outside-in phenomenon, meaning, something outside the body causes it to become ill. Although occasionally necessary for critical health problems, prescription drugs given for chronic conditions are nothing more than suppressive medicine. They eliminate a symptom, but do nothing to correct the underlying *cause* of the problem. Health is defined as being well in the absence of pharmaceuticals; health is *not* defined as the absence of symptoms in the presence of drugs.

Learn the truth about vaccines—the flu shot will not protect you and may have serious consequences in one way or another for many, if not all, who receive it. The bird flu vaccine will lead to an increased risk of serious illness if mixed with the dioxin-influenza combination. Vaccines are not the answer to the bird flu problem for chickens either; in fact, they will only serve to further disrupt the immune system of the birds. Cleaning up the terrain—in humans, in birds, and that of the terra firma—is the answer.

The time has come for everyone to participate. There is no time left for passivity. Each person must step outside his or her comfort zone and get involved; what is happening is both a temporal and a spiritual battle. Everyone here is responsible for the fate of our planet, but those with means have a greater responsibility. Use whatever resources you are blessed to have to get active. If you can't get motivated enough to get engaged for yourself, do it for your children and your grandchildren.

Think of the imperative reasons to engage:
- You have been methodically stripped of your Constitutional and civil rights to refuse mandatory medication and vaccines that may be forced on you and your children by your government. Now, pharma has been handed government protection for even faulty

products.

- Millions of innocent men, women, and children have been bombed and burned by billions of pounds of chemicals and DU.
- Our food supply is being genetically manipulated into commodities that have not been proven safe and may very well be making us sick.
- Animals are being abused and killed mercilessly for profit. The farmers of the world are being systematically turned into serfs, no different than the feudal system of the Dark Ages.

There are 300 million Americans across this great land; there are about 1,000 politicians and bureaucrats in Washington. They are *our* employees. We pay their salaries, and they give themselves outrageous raises and benefit packages, without our permission, that we can't afford to pay. They are stealing from our company— our country—and giving us orders. We should be marching in the streets and they should all be fired.

A call to action

Speaking out is not being a fanatic. George Washington, Thomas Jefferson, and Patrick Henry were all branded extremists and radicals by agents of the British Crown. If your friends label you as such, you are in pretty good company.

We need to make our voices heard. Our representatives must stop wasting our money to develop toxic and ineffective vaccines, stockpile worthless drugs, and give drug companies, chemical companies, and agribusinesses complete liability protection for their destructive products. It is imperative for the citizens of the world and members of diverse activist groups to band together. We must to stop the decimation of the planet and all her inhabitants through the combined effects of global sister businesses and war. Unlike the Puritans and the Pilgrims, who left a society they could no longer tolerate, if the earth's basic resources—soil, water, air, and food— become contaminated beyond use, we have no escape. There is no new continent, no other planet. We must take care of the only one we have. We must to fight to save her.

The distinctions between drug companies, the chemical companies, and agribusiness are razor thin and the boundaries are conspicuously blurred. Governments and WHO officials seem unwilling to indict agribusiness for the adverse health conditions of their domestic fowl, and have given only a cursory nod to the cleanup programs that would decrease health risks for humans and birds alike. The WHO and the FAO would rather blame migratory birds—easy scapegoats. But it should be crystal clear by now that the tens of billions of dollars being squandered on special interest groups should be allocated to environmental groups who are involved with cleaning up the planet, protecting our food supply, and restoring our health without drugs.

The exorbitant amount of money being used to fight "wars without end" should be reassigned to the development of renewable, environmentally friendly resources. Instead of spending hundreds of millions of dollars each year to wipe out the last vestiges of the polio virus in remote villages in Africa, funds should be committed to teaching hygiene, building safe homes, providing farmers with non-genetically modified grain, and digging wells for potable water. Allocating resources for projects to help the world's poorest inhabitants would improve the planet for decades to come. Without a combined, worldwide cleanup effort and adequate human detoxification programs, the pandemic will surely occur at some point in the future.[10]

But not for the reasons you are being told.

WHAT YOU CAN DO

This is a very limited list of the many organization that deserve your support and your time.

United Poultry Concerns, Inc.
Karen Davis, PhD, President
PO Box 150
Machipongo, VA 23405-0150
757-678-7875
Fax: 757-678-5070
www.upc-online.org

Environmental Working Group (EWG)
Environmental Working Group, founded in 1993, brings to light unsettling facts, spotlights shameful activity of polluters and their lobbyists, and rattles politicians who shape policy. EWG reviews produces investigations on toxic chemicals, farm subsidies, public lands, and other topics and earns regular coverage from media outlets nationwide.
Washington, D.C. Headquarters
1436 U Street NW, Suite 100
Washington, DC 20009
202-667-6982
Fax: 202-232-2592

www.ewg.org

WWF *(formerly World Wildlife Fund)*
In just over four decades, WWF has become one of the world's largest and most respected independent conservation organizations.
U.S. Headquarters
WWF
1250 24th Street, N.W.
P.O. Box 97180
Washington, D.C. 20090-7180
202-293-4800
www.worldwildlife.org

A GUIDE TO BIOMONITORING OF INDUSTRIAL CHEMICALS

This is a guidebook about human biomonitoring—the measurement of chemicals in human tissue—that brings together many information resources, organizes them by topic area, and provides a brief annotated description of each. The goal is to help you select resources relevant to your concern. Online, the chapters are connected electronically to the table of contents for easy use.

Center for Children's Health and the Environment Department of Community and Preventive Medicine
Box 1043
Mount Sinai School of Medicine
New York, NY 10029
212-241-8806
Fax: 212-360-6965
Email: christopher.oleskey@mssm.edu

GOVERNMENT ORGANIZATIONS

ACIP: The Advisory Committee on Immunization Practices consists of 15 experts selected by the head of the Department of Health and Human Services. The committee develops written recommendations for the routine administration of vaccines to the pediatric and adult populations, along with schedules regarding the appropriate periodicity, dosage, and contraindications applicable to the vaccines. ACIP is the only entity in the federal government that makes such recommendations.

The overall goals of the ACIP are to provide guidance that will assist the department and the nation in reducing the incidence of vaccine-preventable diseases and to increase the safe usage of vaccines and related biological products.
(http://www.cdc.gov/nip/ ACIP/ default.htm.)

ATSDR: The Agency for Toxic Substances and Disease Registry is part of the U.S. Department of Health and Human Services and is the principal federal public health agency involved with hazardous waste issues. ATSDR is responsible for preventing or reducing the harmful effects of exposure to hazardous substances on human health and quality of life.

CBER: The Center for Biologics Evaluation and Research is a division of the FDA. CBER regulates the licensing of vaccines and other biological products. CBER and the CDC jointly manage the Vaccine Adverse Event Reporting System (VAERS).
(http://www.fda.gov/cber.)

CDC: Centers for Disease Control is one of the 13 major operating components of the Department of Health and Human Services (HHS)—the principal agency in the United States government created for the protection of the health and safety of all Americans.
(http://www.cdc.gov.)

251

EPA: The Environmental Protection Agency's mission is to protect human health and the environment. Since 1970, the EPA has been working for a cleaner, healthier environment for the American people. It is charged with the regulation of pesticides in the U.S. by a system of registration and review. The administrator of the EPA is appointed by the president. (http://www.epa.gov/.)

FDA: The Food and Drug Administration is the federal agency responsible for ensuring that foods are safe, wholesome, and sanitary; human and veterinary drugs, biological products, and medical devices are safe and effective; cosmetics are safe; and electronic products that emit radiation are safe. According to the FDA Web site, it is the role of the FDA to ensure that these products are "honestly, accurately, and informatively represented to the public." (http://www.fda.gov.)

HEW: The Department of Health, Education, and Welfare was a cabinet level department of the U.S. government from 1953 until 1979. In 1979, a separate Department of Education was created from this department, and HEW was renamed the Department of Health and Human Services.

DHHS: The Department of Health and Human Services is sometimes listed only as HHS. This is a Cabinet department of the U.S. government. The secretary of HHS is appointed by the president. In 2004, HHS registered 67,000 employees and had a combined mandatory and discretionary budget of $640.7 billion.

IOM: The Institutes of Medicine is part of the National Academy of Sciences. The Institute is charged with providing unbiased, evidence-based, and authoritative information and advice concerning health and science policy to policy-makers, professionals, leaders in every sector of society, and the public at large. (http://www.iom.edu/.)

IPEN: Founded in 1998, the International POPs Elimination Network is a global network of public interest and non-governmental organizations (NGOs) united in support of a common goal. The mission of IPEN is to work for the global elimination of persistent organic pollutants on an expeditious yet socially equitable basis.

NIBSC: The National Institute of Biological Standards and Control is the FDA equivalent in the UK. NIBSC is a laboratory-based organization with special expertise in quality control and standardization of the biological products used in medicine in the U.K. (http://www.nibsc.ac.uk/.)

NIAID: The National Institute of Allergy and Infectious Diseases (NIAID) conducts and supports basic and applied research to better understand, treat, and ultimately prevent infectious, immunologic, and allergic diseases. Anthony S. Fauci, MD, has been director of NIAID since 1984 and is responsible for the proposed fiscal year 2006 budget of approximately $4.4 billion.
(http://www3.niaid.nih.gov/.)

WHO: The World Health Organization is the United Nations' specialized agency for health, established in 1948. The WHO's stated objective is "the attainment by all peoples of the highest possible level of health." The WHO is governed by 192 member states through the World Health Assembly. The Health Assembly is composed of representatives from WHO's member states who approve WHO programs and its annual budget.
(http://www.who.int.)

VRBPAC: The Vaccines and Related Biological Products Advisory Committee is a division within the FDA that first reviews new vaccines and vaccine applications.

GLOSSARY

ADI: Acceptable Daily Intake. The amount of a particular chemical in food that can be consumed on a daily basis over a lifetime without harm. An assumption made by the EPA, WHO, etc., based on data from a variety of sources including laboratory testing.

Adventitious: Accidentally added from the outside; not inherent; occurring in abnormal places. As in vaccines, an adventitious virus is an "extra virus" that was not intended to be part of the formulation.

Antigen: A substance that is foreign to the body and stimulates the immune system to produce antibodies. Antigens include foreign proteins, bacteria, viruses, pollen, and other materials. The influenza viral surface proteins (H) and (N) are antigens.

Body Burden: The total amount of a chemical stored in the body at a given time.

CP: The poultry powerhouse in Southeast Asia—the Bangkok-based Charoen Pokphand (CP). A multinational conglomerate employing more than 100,000 people in 20 countries. CP's core business is food production.

Cytokine: A protein produced by white blood cells, particularly NK and CD8+ cells, in the presence of viral infections. Cytokines act as chemical messengers between cells, initiating a cascade of events to eliminate the foreign microorganism from the body.

cDNA: The DNA that is made by reverse transcriptase from RNA. The normal flow of genetic replication is from DNA to RNA; when this happens in reverse, it is represented as cDNA.

DNA: The basic material of a cell that contains the genetic code and transmits hereditary patterns.

Dioxin: Dioxin is a general term that describes a complex family of more than 400 chemicals that are highly persistent in the environment. It is an unintentional waste product formed during industrial processes that use chlorine. Incineration of plastics, pesticide manufacturing and paper bleaching all result in the production of dioxin.

Gene: A part of the DNA that represents a fundamental unit of heredity. Most genes create proteins for use in the cell.

GBS: Guillain-Barré syndrome. An inflammatory disorder of the peripheral nerves (those outside the brain and spinal cord). Called an "ascending paralysis," GBS starts in the legs and moves up the body, quickly involving the muscles that aid in breathing (including the diaphragm), resulting in respiratory failure. Maximal muscle weakness typically occurs two weeks after the onset of symptoms, and treatment often involves long-term, intensive care hospitalization, with most patients needing the assistance of a respirator.

HPAI: Highly Pathogenic Avian Influenza viruses. Influenza type A viruses that have been reported to cause widespread mortality among the bird population. All outbreaks of HPAI since the 1980s have been caused by surface antigen subtypes H5 or H7. Human infections have also occurred in the presence of the H9 antigen, but at this time, this protein considered highyly pathogenic. The bird flu virus, H5N1, is considered to be a HPAI virus.

Homeostasis: Maintenance of the body's internal environment in balance; the condition in which the body's internal environment remains relatively constant to optimize physiological functions.

Mitosis: The process of cellular division in cells that produces daughter cells genetically identical to each other and to the parent cell.

Molecular Mimicry: A phenomenon associated with some pathogens, where the surface proteins of the pathogen are very similar to the surface proteins in the body. In the absence of the pathogen (virus or bacteria), the antibody, often induced by a vaccine, can attack the surface protein of the body. The result is an autoimmune reaction, such as in rheumatoid arthritis or lupus.

Normal Flora: Bacteria, fungi, and protozoa that live on or within the bodies of animals and plants. By definition, organisms that are part of an animal's normal flora do not cause disease in healthy individuals and can even be beneficial. Acidophilus and lactobacillus are two examples.

Oncogene: A gene capable of causing the transformation of normal cells into cancer cells. The oncogene can be activated by a virus.

Pandemic: A disease outbreak impacting a large geographical area, crossing international boundaries and usually affecting a large number of people.

Parts per trillion (ppt): An expression of the concentration of a chemical per trillion units of the medium in which it is being measured (e.g., blood or water). Larger concentrations may be parts per thousand. Can be expressed as ng/kg.

Pharma: Short for "pharmaceutical industry."

POPs: Persistent Organic Pollutants. Chemicals named by the Swedish Convention to be eliminated from the planet and called the "Dirty Dozen" include aldrin, chlordane, DDT, dieldrin, endrin, heptachlor, mirex, toxaphene, hexachlorobenzene, polychlorinated biphenyls, dioxins, and furans.

Proto-oncogene: A normal cellular gene that can be transformed into an active oncogene. The conversion can be caused by mutation, DNA rearrangement, or nearby insertion of viral DNA into a gene.

Reference Dose (RfD): Defined by the EPA as "an estimate of a daily exposure to the human population that is likely to be without an appreciable risk of deleterious (harmful) effects during a lifetime."

RNA: A single-strand of nucleic acid. There are many forms of RNA, including messenger RNA, transfer RNA, and ribosomal RNA. All types can be involved with protein synthesis and viral replication.

Specific-pathogen free (SPF): A term used to designate cell cultures and tissues (such as eggs) used to grow viruses for vaccines that have been tested for a specific list of organisms with a specific set of tests/methods used to detect the organisms. While SPF means the cultures do not contain the organisms tested for, it does not mean that the substrate is free of all pathogens.

Serology testing: A type of testing done on the serum in the blood (the clear portion of the blood without the cells) to identify certain proteins, such as an antibody. When exposed to a microorganism, such as a virus, the body produces specific antibodies against it. In laboratory testing, the antibodies react with antigens in specific ways to confirm the identity or presence of a microorganism; this test is not used to diagnose a current infection.

Symbiont: An organism that coexists with another organism in a mutually beneficial relationship. Example: the bacteria that live in the intestinal tract or vaginal cavity in humans.

TDI: Tolerable Daily Intake. An estimate of the quantity of a chemical contaminant that can be ingested in food every day over a lifetime without posing a significant risk to health.

TEF: A toxic equivalency factor (TEF) is assigned to each dioxin based on its potency compared to TCDD.

TEQ(s): Toxic Equivalents. A value is assigned to each dioxin and dioxin-like compound by the EPA that is a comparison to the most toxic dioxin, TCDD. When several compounds are released together, the TEQ is the combined toxicity.

Toxicity: The capacity of a chemical to have a specific adverse effect on an organism. The toxicity of a chemical includes its potency—the strength of the chemical per unit of exposure.

Virulent: Description of an organism considered to be extremely poisonous, injurious, or deadly and able to violently and rapidly overcome the natural defenses of the host. Said of an organism that is highly infectious.

260

ENDNOTES

CHAPTER 1: THINKING FOR YOURSELF

1 (Baker, Frank W. "Thirty Second Ad Cost," *Math in the Media*, Media Literacy Clearinghouse, 27 September 2004.
(http://medialit.med.sc.edu/thirtysecadcosts.htm.)
2 Nowak, Glen PhD. "Planning for the 2004–05 Influenza Vaccination Season: A Communication Situation Analysis," American Medical Association.
(http://www.ama-assn.org/ama1/pub/upload/mm/36/2004_flu_nowak.pdf .)
3 Lewandowsky, Stephan, et al. "Memory for Fact, Fiction, and Misinformation," *Psychological Science* 16 (3), 190–195, 2005.
4 Begley, Sharon. "People Believe a 'Fact' That Fits Their Views Even if It's Clearly False," *The Wall Street Journal* B1, 4 February 2005.
5 Lewandowsky, Stephan. "Misinformation: Seeing Is Believing," *American* Psychological Society, 17 May 2005. (http://www.psychologicalscience.org/media/releases/2005/pr050517.cfm.)
6 Rosenthal, Elisabeth. "2 Studies Question the Effectiveness of Flu Vaccines," *The New York Times*, 21 September 2005.
7 Van Essen, G. A., Palache, A. M., Forleo, E., Fedson, D. S. "Influenza vaccination in 2000: recommendations and vaccine use in 50 developed and rapidly developing countries," *Vaccine*, Vol. 21, Issue 16 (2003): pp. 1780–1785.

CHAPTER 2: THE FLU AS WE KNOW IT

1 Koehler, Christopher S. W. "History of plagues" condensed from "Camp Followers," *Modern Drug Discovery* 4 (2001).
2 Billings, Molly. *The Influenza Pandemic of 1918*. Stanford, Calif.: Stanford University, June 1997.

CHAPTER 3: THE AVIAN FLU: WHAT YOU NEED TO KNOW

1 Fouchier, R. A. "Characterization of a novel influenza A virus hemagglutinin subtype (H16) obtained from black-headed gulls," *Journal of Virology* 79 (2005): 14–22.
2 Duke University PowerPoint presentation available online at http://duke.usask.ca/~misra/virology/slides/flu.ppt#272,11,Nomenclature.Slide #11.
3 "Taxonomy Browser." National Center for Biotechnology Information.
(http://www.ncbi.nlm.nih.gov/Taxonomy/ Browser.
4 Russell, Sabin, Holding, Reynolds, Fernandez, Elizabeth. "Breakdowns Mar Flu Shot Program Production, distribution delays raise fears of nation vulnerable to epidemic," *San Francisco Chronicle*, 25 February 2001, p. A1.
5 Sen, Sumit K. "Avian Influenza (or Bird Flu) and India," *The Birds of Kolkata*.
(http://www.kolkatabirds.com/birdflu.htm).
6 Clark, Dustan F., MD. "Avian Influenza, always a threat in the fall," University

of Arkansas, Fall 2000. Vol. 2. No. 1.
(http://www.uark.edu/depts/posc/avian_advice_vol2.1.pdf.)
[7] "Hong Kong orders poultry slaughter," BBC News, 18 May 2001.
(http://news.bbc.co.uk/1/hi/world/asia-pacific/1337414.stm.)
[8] "Interim Recommendations for Persons with Possible Exposure to Avian
Influenza During Outbreaks Among Poultry in the United States," The Centers for
Disease Control and Prevention. (http://www.cdc.gov).
[9] Borgeois, Ricky. "Avian influenza found in non-commercial, commercial
Delaware flocks," *American Farm Publications, Inc.*, 7 February 2004.
(http://www.americanfarm.com/Poultry2-17-04a.html.)
[10] TABLE 1: WHO. "Avian influenza A(H5N1)–update 31: Situation (poultry) in
Asia: for a long-term response, comparison with previous outbreaks." World
Health Organization. 2 March 2004.
(http://www.who.int/csr/don/2004_03_02/en/.) *(Reproduced with permission from
the WHO.)*
[11] (http://duke.usask.ca/~misra/virology/slides/flu.ppt#289,15,Reassortment.)
[12] Wong, Derek. "Influenza Viruses," Virology-Online. (http://virology-
online.com/viruses/Influenza.htm.)
[13] Niman, Henry L. "1933 Sequences in 2004 Korean H1N1 Swine Isolates Raise
Concern," *Recombinomics*, 22 December 2004.
[14] Gibbs, M. J., Armstrong, J. S., Gibbs, A. J. "The haemagglutinin gene, but not the
neuraminidase gene, of 'Spanish flu' was a recombinant." *Philosophical Transactions
of the Royal Society of London* 365 (2001): 1845–1855.
[15] Kolata, Gina. "Experts Unlock Clues to Spread of 1918 Flu Virus," *The New York
Times*, 6 October 2005. (http://www.nytimes.com.)

CHAPTER 4: PERSPECTIVE: PAST PANDEMICS

[1] Yuen, K.Y., Wong. S. S. Y. "Human infection by avian influenza A H5N1," *Hong
Kong Medical Journal*, June 2005.
(http://www.hkam.org.hk/publications/hkmj/article_pdfs/hkm0506p189.pdf.)
[2] World Health Organization Writing Group. "Nonpharmaceutical Interventions
for Pandemic Influenza, National and Community Measures," *Emerging Infectious
Diseases* 12 (2006). (http://www.cdc.gov/ncidod/EID/vol12no01/05-1371.htm.)
[3] Milloy, Steven. "Flu Proposal Misguided," Nov.3, 2005. Fox News Report.
(http://www.foxnews.com/story/0.2933.174521.00.html.)
[4] Noymer, Andrew and Garenne, Michel. "The 1918 Influenza Epidemic's Efects
on Sex Differentials in Mortality in the United States," Population and
Development Review. 26(3):565-581. September 2000.
[5] "Transcript of Press Briefing Pandemic Influenza Plan," U.S. Department of
Health and Human Services, 2 November 2005.
(http://www.hhs.gov/news/transcripts/briefing20051102.html.)
[6] "Avian influenza: assessing the pandemic threat," World Health Organization,
January 2005. (http://www.who.int/csr/disease/influenza/H5N1-9reduit.pdf.)
[7] "Avian influenza: assessing the pandemic threat," World Health Organization,

January 2005. (http://www.who.int/csr/disease/influenza/H5N1-9reduit.pdf, p. 32.)

8 "If It's Not HIV, What Can Cause AIDS?" *Alive & Well AIDS Alternatives* (http://www.aliveandwell.org/ html/ if_its_not/ifitsnothiv.html).

9 "Avian influenza: assessing the pandemic threat," World Health Organization, January 2005. (http://www.who.int/csr/disease/influenza/H5N1-9reduit.pdf p. 32.)

10 "Prevention of Plague," Recommendations of the Advisory Committee on Immunization Practices, The Centers for Disease Control and Prevention, 13 December 1996. (http://www.cdc.gov/mmwr/PDF/rr/rr4514.pdf.)

CHAPTER 5: RECENT FIASCOS: THE SWINE FLU AND THE SMALLPOX SCARE

1 Warner, Joel. "The Sky is Falling: An Analysis of the Swine Flu Affair of 1976," Haverford College. (http://www.haverford.edu/biology/edwards/disease/viral_essays/ warnervirus.htm.)

2 Schmeck, Harold M. "U.S. Calls Flu Alert on Possible Return of Epidemic Virus," *The New York Times,* 20 February 1976, p. 69.

3 After leaving Congress in 1979, Rep. Rogers became a member of the Board of Directors for Merck & Co. and Mutual Life Insurance of New York.

4 Russell, Sabin. "When polio vaccine backfired: Tainted batches killed 10 and paralyzed 164," *San Francisco Chronicle,* 25 April 2005, p. A1.

5 Swine Flu Act. Pub. L. 94-380; 42 U.S.C. 247b(j)-(l) (1976).

6 Neustadt, Richard E., Fineberg, Harvey, V. "The Swine Flu Affair: Decision-making on a Slippery Disease," DHEW, 1978.

7 Neustadt, Richard E., Fineberg, Harvey, V. "The Swine Flu Affair: Decision-making on a Slippery Disease," DHEW, 1978 (excerpt), LSU Law Center's Medical and Public Health Law Site.

8 Kent, Christopher, MD. "Flu Shots," *The Chiropractic Journal* (May 2000). (http://www.worldchiropracticalliance.org/tcj/2000/may/may2000kent.htm.)

9 Fanion, David. "Guillain-Barré Syndrome," *EMedicine*, 14 August 2004. (http://www.emedicine.com/EMERG/topic222.htm.)

10 Neustadt, Richard E., Fineberg, Harvey, V. "The Swine Flu Affair: Decision-making on a Slippery Disease," DHEW (1978).

11 Liability for Swine Flu Vaccine – Unthank v. United States, 732 F.2d 1517 (10th Cir. 1984). LSU Law Center's Medical and Public Health Law Site. (http://biotech.law.lsu.edu/cases/vaccines/Unthank.htm.)

12 Krasner, Gary. "Another Bipartisan Multi-Billion Dollar Medical Boondoggle: How Biomedical Research Takes Congress And Our Money, Part 1, " *The American Daily*, 29 July 2004. (http://www.americandaily.com/article/4469.)

13 "One Hundred Heroes and Icons of the 20th Century," *Time Magazine*, June 14, 1999.

14 Neustadt, Richard E., Fineberg, Harvey, V. "The Swine Flu Affair: Decision-making on a Slippery Disease," DHEW, 1978.

15 Working Group on Civilian Biodefense. "Smallpox as a Biological Weapon Medical and Public Health Management," *Journal of the American Medical Association*

(JAMA) 281 (1999): 2127–2137.

16 "Vaccinia (Smallpox) Vaccine Recommendations of the Advisory Committee on Immunization Practices (ACIO)," *Morbidity and Mortality Weekly Report* (MMWR), June 22, 2001 /50(RR10); 1–25).

17 (Emphasis added.) Beigel, J. H. "Avian influenza A(H5N1) infection in humans," *New England Journal of Medicine* 353 (2005):1374–85.

18 World Health Organization International Avian Influenza Investigative Team. "Avian influenza A(H5N1) in 10 patients in Vietnam," *New England Journal Medicine* 350 (2004):1179–1188.

19 World Health Organization International Avian Influenza Investigative Team. "Lack of H5N1 avian influenza transmission to hospital employees," *Emerging Infectious Diseases* 11 (2005): 210–215.

20 Ungchusak, K. et al. "Probable person-to-person transmission of avian influenza A(H5N1)," *New England Journal of Medicine* 352 (2005): 333–340.

21 MMWR. Achievements in Public Health, 1900-1999 Impact of Vaccines Universally recommended for children–United States, 1990-1998. April 02, 1999 / 78(12);243-248

22 Adler, Jerry. "The Fight Against The Flu," *Newsweek*, 39–45, October 31, 2005.

23 Roos, Robert. "Relatives of avian flu patients have asymptomatic cases," CIDRAP News, 9 March 2005.

24 Paulos, John Allen. "Who's Counting: Flu Deaths, Iraqi Dead Numbers Skewed," ABC News.

25 Del Giudice, G., Podda, A., Rappuoli, R. "What are the limits of adjuvanticity?" *Vaccine* 20 (2001): S38–S41.

26 "Notice to Readers: Considerations for Distinguishing Influenza-Like Illness from Inhalational Anthrax," *Morbidity and Mortality Weekly Report (MMWR)*, 9 November 2001. (http://www.cdc.gov/mmwr/preview/mmwrhtml/mm5044a5.htm.)

27 "Secretary Thompson to Release $100 Million to Assist States with Smallpox Vaccination Programs," U.S. Department of Health & Human Services, 5 May 2003. (http://www.hhs.gov/news/press/2003pres/20030505a.html.)

28 Source: Neustadt, PhD, Richard E., Fineberg, MD, PhD, Harvey, V. "The Swine Flu Affair: Decision-making on a Slippery Disease," DHEW, 1978. Dr. Fineberg is a past-president of the Institute of Medicine.

Chapter 6: The New Play Book Arrives

1 Nowak, Glen PhD "Planning for the 2004–05 Influenza Vaccination Season: A Communication Situation Analysis," American Medical Association. (http://www.ama-assn.org/ama1/pub/upload/mm/36/2004_flu_nowak.pdf Full document can be read at www.NoMercury.org

2 "SARS fatalities." NationMaster.com: (http://www.nationmaster.com/graph-T/hea_sar_fat.)

3 Osterholm, Michael. "Preparing for the Next Pandemic," *Foreign Affairs*, July/August 2005.

4 "SARS hits Singapore Air's Bottom Line," *BizAsia,* 30 August 2003.

5 Jong-wook, Lee, Director General. "Meeting on avian influenza and pandemic human influenza," World Health Organization, 7 November 2005. (http://www.who.int/dg/lee/speeches/2005/flupandemicgeneva/en/.)

6 Osterholm, Michael. "Preparing for the Next Pandemic," *Foreign Affairs,* July/August 2005.

7 Sandman, Peter and Lanard, Jody. Bird Flu: "Communicating the Risks," *Perspectives in Health,* 10 (2005). (http://www.paho.org/english/DD/PIN/Number22_article1.htm.)

8 Hirschman, Dave. "CDC chief treads lightly with flu news," *The Atlanta Journal-Constitution,* October 20, 2005. (http//www.aja.com.)

9 Sandman, Peter and Lanard, Jody. Bird Flu: "Communicating the Risks," *Perspectives in Health* 10 (2005). (http://www.paho.org.)

CHAPTER 7: VACCINES: A SHORT SUMMARY OF A LONG HISTORY

1 A complete review of the history of the vaccination is far beyond the scope of this text. For more information, consider the book *Bodily Matters* by Nadja Durbach (2005). Older books such as *Vaccines and Evil Serum* by Herbert M. Shelton (1935) and *The Case Against Vaccination* by Dr. Walter Hadwen (1896) are extremely interesting recounts of the early use of the smallpox vaccine. A collection of well-written historical observations on the history of smallpox and other vaccines are available on CD through Vaccine Liberation, at http//www.vaclib.org.

2 Transcript of ACIP meeting in Atlanta, Georgia, June 19 and 20, 2002.

3 Walsh, David and Whyte, Alan. "U.S. officials debate how to ration flu vaccine," World Socialist Web Site, 1 November 2004.

4 "Best of What's New Showcase," *Popular Science,* November 2003.

5 "Nasal spray for flu to get big media launch," *The Washington Post E01,* 10 September 2003.

6 Madjid, Mohammed. "Influenza as a bioweapon," *Journal of the Royal Society of Medicine 96* (2003): 345–346.

7 Kwiatkowski, Holly. "A Seat at the Table," *Contingencies,* October 2005.

CHAPTER 8: INFLUENZA VACCINES: WHAT'S IN THAT NEEDLE

1 Spotswood, Stephen. "NIAID Researching, Predicting The Future Of Flu," *U.S. Medicine,* December 2004. (http://www.usmedicine.com/article.cfm?articleID=996&issueID=69.)

2 "WHO manual on animal influenza diagnosis and surveillance," World Health Organization, 1 September 2004. (http://www.who.int/csr/resources/publications/influenza/WHO_CDS_CSR_NCS_2002_5/en/.)

3 "Octyphenol Ethoxylate," The Dow Chemical Company. (http://www.dow.com.)

4 "Influenza Virus Vaccine Fluzone 2005–2006 Formula," package insert. Aventis Pasteur (company name has since changed to Sanofi Pasteur MSD. Update 14 February 2006).

[5] Gray, S., Demicheli, V., Di Pietrantonj, C., Harnden, A. R., Jefferson, T., Matheson, N. J., Rivetti, A. "Vaccines for preventing influenza in healthy children," *The Cochrane Database of Systematic Reviews* 1 (2006).

[6] Kennedy, Laura. "Flu Shots for Toddlers Not Backed By Evidence, Major Study Says," *Health Behavior News Service*, 24 January 2006.

[7] Carey, Elaine. "Flu shot for tots slammed by study," *Toronto Star*, 27 Jan. 2006, 21:37:17.

[8] Demicheli, V., Rivetti, D., Deeks, J. J., Jefferson, T. O. "Vaccines for preventing influenza in healthy adults," *The Cochrane Database of Systematic Reviews*, 1 (2006)

[9] Data sheet acquired directly from Charles River Laboratories, headquartered near Boston, MA, is a developer of specific pathogen-free fertilized chicken eggs used in poultry vaccines. (www.criver.com.)

[10] Press Release. "Federal Guidelines Needed to Ensure Safety in Animal-to-Human Organ Transplants," National Academy of Sciences, 17 July 17 1996. (http://www4.nas.edu/news.nsf/isbn/0309055490?OpenDocument.)

[11] Norman, J. E., Gilbert, W. B., Jay, H. H., Leonard, B. S. "Mortality follow-up of the 1942 epidemic of hepatitis B in the U.S. Arm," *Hepatology* 18 (1993): 790–797.

[12] For a full discussion on the contamination of the polio vaccines with SV40, see the book by Debbie Bookchin and Jim Schumacher, *The Virus and the Vaccine: The True Story of a Cancer-Causing Monkey Virus, Contaminated Polio Vaccine, and the Millions of Americans Exposed*, St. Martin's Press, 2004.

[13] "Evolving Scientific and Regulatory Perspectives on cell substrates for vaccine development," Food and Drug Administration, Center for Biologics Evaluation and Research, 10 September 1999. (http://www.fda.gov/cber/minutes/0910evolv.txt.)

[14] (Charles River Laboratory Chart used with permission by Charles River Labs. It is a representative chart of viruses that are tested to create pathogen-specific eggs.)

[15] Felder, M. P., Eychene, A., Laugier, D., Marx, M., Dezelee, P., Calothy, G. "Steps and mechanisms of oncogene transduction by retroviruses," *Folia Biologica (Praha)*, 40 (1994): 225–235.

[16] "Evolving Scientific and Regulatory Perspectives on cell substrates for vaccine development," Food and Drug Administration, Center for Biologics Evaluation and Research, 10 September 1999. http://www.fda.gov/cber/ minutes/ 0910evolv .txt.)

[17] Weiss, R. *RNA tumor viruses*, New York: Cold Spring Harbor Laboratory Press; 1982. pp. 1109–1203.

[18] Shirley X. Tsang, William M. Switzer, Vedapuri Shanmugam, Jeffrey A. Johnson, Cynthia Goldsmith, Anthony Wright, Aly Fadly, Donald Thea, Harold Jaffe, Thomas M. Folks, and Walid Heneine. Evidence of Avian Leukosis Virus Subgroup E and Endogenous Avian Virus in Measles and Mumps Vaccines Derived from Chicken Cells: Investigation of Transmission to Vaccine Recipients. J Virol. 1999 July; 73(7): 5843–5851.

[19] "Concerns about Vaccine Contamination," The Centers for Disease Control and Prevention. (http://www.cdc.gov/nip/vacsafe/concerns/gen/contamination.htm.)

[20] "Evolving Scientific and Regulatory Perspectives on cell substrates for vaccine

development," Food and Drug Administration, Center for Biologics Evaluation and Research, 10 September 1999. (http://www.fda.gov/cber/minutes/0910evolv.txt.)

[21] Alberts, Bray, Johnson, Lewis, Raff, Roberts, and Walter. "The Life Cycle Of A Retrovirus," Garland Publishing (1998).

[22] McRearden, Benjamin. "What Is Coming Through That Needle? The Problem of Pathogenic Vaccine Contamination," Townsend Letter, October (2003).

[23] Epstein, Samuel and Young, Quentin, MD. "Escalating Incidence of Childhood Cancer Ignored," Environmental News Service, 9 May 2002. (http://www.ens-newswire.com/ens/may2002/2002-05-09e.aspAlberts.)

[24] Epstein, Samuel and Young, Quentin, MD.[23]

[25] "Evolving Scientific and Regulatory Perspectives on Cell Substrates for Vaccine Development," Center for Biologics Evaluation and Research, 10 September 1999. (http://www.fda.gov/cber/minutes/0910evolv.txt.)

[26] "Evolving Scientific and Regulatory Perspectives on Cell Substrates for Vaccine Development," Center for Biologics Evaluation and Research, 10 September 1999. (http://www.fda.gov/cber/minutes/0910evolv.txt.)

[27] "Evolving Scientific and Regulatory Perspectives on Cell Substrates for Vaccine Development," Center for Biologics Evaluation and Research, 10 Sept. 1999. (http://www.fda.gov/cber/minutes/0910evolv.txt.)

[28] Weissmahr, R. N., Schupbach, J., Boni, J. "Reverse transcriptase activity in chicken embryo fibroblast culture supernatants is associated with particles containing endogenous avian retrovirus EAV-0 RNA," *Journal of Virology* 71 (1997): 3005–3012.

Chapter 9: Beyond Eggs: Cell-Culture Vaccines and Toxic Adjuvants

[1] MacKenzie, Debora. "US flu vaccine trials may be effort wasted," *New Scientist*, 25 March 2005. (http://www.newscientist.com/article.ns?id=dn7172.)

[2] MacKenzie, Debora. "Low-dose bird flu vaccine tested on humans," *New Scientist*, 16 Sept. 2005. (http://www.newscientist.com/article.ns?id=dn8009.)

[3] Beigel, J. H. "Avian influenza A(H5N1) infection in humans," *New England Journal of Medicine* 353 (2005):1374–85.

[4] "New Sanofi plant increases vaccine production," *in-Pharma Technologist*, 21 July 2005. (http://www.in-pharmatechnologist.com.)

[5] Ref. No. 1: Govorkova, E. A., Kaverin, N. V., Gubareva, L. V., Meignier, B., Webster, R.G. "Replication of influenza A viruses in a green monkey kidney continuous cell line (Vero)," *The Journal of Infectious Diseases* 172 (1995): 250–253. Ref. No. 2: Govorkova, E. A., Murti, G., Meignier, B., de Taisne, C., Webster, R.G. "African green monkey kidney (Vero) cells provide an alternative host cell system for influenza A and B viruses," *Journal of Virology* 70 (1996): 5519–5524.

[6] For full information see the paper published by Carbone and Risso, "Simian virus 40, polio vaccines and human tumors: a review of recent developments," *Oncogene* 15 (1997): 1877–1888. The tumors were ependymomas and choroid plexus tumors (brain tissue); mesothelioma (lung tissue); and osteosarcomas and sarcomas (bone tissue).

[7] For the complete, well-written discussion regarding the polio vaccine, SV40, and Dr. Carbone's work, see the book by Debbie Bookchin and Jim Schumacher, *The Virus and the Vaccine: The True Story of a Cancer-Causing Monkey Virus, Contaminated Polio Vaccine, and the Millions of Americans Exposed* (St. Martin's Press, 2004). For a family's story and condensed information on SV40, go to http//www.SV40Foundation.org.

[8] Midthun, Karen, MD. "Letter to Sponsors Using Vero Cells as a Cell Substrate for Investigational Vaccines." Food and Drug Administration, Center for Biologics Evaluation and Research, 12 March 2001.
(http://www.fda.gov/cber/ltr/vero031301.htm.)

[9] "Baxter Suspends Enrollment in European Clinical Trial for PreFluCel," Baxter, 9 December 2004.

[10] "?'Designer' Cells as Substrates for the Manufacture of Viral Vaccines," Food and Drug Administration.
(http://www.fda.gov/ohrms/dockets/ac/01/briefing/3750b1_01.htm.)

[11] "Influenza Vaccines under development," Protein Sciences Corporation.
(http://www.proteinsciences.com/vaccines.htm#rha.)

[12] "Designer" Cells as Substrates for the Manufacture of Viral Vaccines," FDA.
(http://www.fda.gov/ohrms/dockets/ac/01/briefing/3750b1_01.htm.)

[13] Ibid.

[14] Vorberg, I., Raines, A., Story, B., Priola, S. A. "Susceptibility of common fibroblast cell lines to transmissible spongiform encephalopathy agents," *Journal of Infectious Diseases* 189 (2004): 431–439. PMID: 14745700

[15] "Secretary Thompson to Release $100 Million to Assist States with Smallpox Vaccination Programs," United States Department of Health & Human Services, 5 May 2003. (http://www.hhs.gov/news/press/2003pres/20030505a.html.)

[16] Kenney, R. T., Edleman, R. "Survey of human-use adjuvants," *Expert Review of Vaccines* 2 (2) (2003): 167–188.

[17] Kenney, R. T., Edleman, R. "Survey of human-use adjuvants," *Expert Review of Vaccines* 2 (2003): 167–188.

[18] Ibid.

[19] Ibid., p.171.

[20] Ibid.

[21] Matsumoto, Gary. Vaccine A: The Covert Government Experiment That's Killing Our Soldiers and Why GIs Are Only the First Victims Vaccine, 54 (New York: Basic Books).

[22] "United States Patent 6299884. "Adjuvant formulation comprising a submicron oil droplet emulsion," *Patent Storm*, 9 October 2001.
(http://www.patentstorm.us/patents/6299884.html.)

[23] Matsumoto, Gary. 54–5.

[24] Ref. No. 1: Svelander, L., Holm, B. C., Buchtt, A., Lorentzen, J. C., Svelander, L. "Responses of the rat immune system to arthritogenic adjuvant oil," *Scandinavian Journal of Immunology* 54 (2001): 599–605. PMID: 11902335.
Ref. No. 2: Satoh, M., Kuroda, Y., Yoshida, H., Behney, K. M., Mizutani, A., Akaogi, J., Nacionales, D. C., Lorenson, T. D., Rosenbauer, R. J., Reeves, W. H. "Induction of lupus autoantibodies by adjuvants," *Journal of Autoimmunity*, August 21(1) (2003): 1–9.

[25] Coors, Esther A., Seybold, Heidi, Merk, Hans, Mahler, Vera. "Polysorbate 80 in medical products and nonimmunologic anaphylactoid reactions," *Annals of Allergy, Asthma and Immunology* 95 (2005): 593–599.

[26] "Recommendations Contraindications Guide to Contraindications to Vaccinations," The Centers for Disease Control and Prevention. (http://www.cdc.gov/nip/recs/contraindications.htm.)

[27] Del Giudice, G., Podda, A., Rappuoli, R. "What are the limits of adjuvanticity?" *Vaccine* 20 (2001): S38–S41. PMID: 11587808.

[28] Frey, S., Poland, G., Percell, S., Podda, A. "Comparison of the safety, tolerability, and immunogenicity of a MF59-adjuvanted influenza vaccine and a non-adjuvanted influenza vaccine in non-elderly adults," *Vaccine* 21 (2003): 4234–4237. PMID: 14505903.

[29] Podda, A., Del Giudice, G. "MF59-adjuvanted vaccines: increased immunogenicity with an optimal safety profile," *Expert Review of Vaccines* 2 (2003): 197-204, p. 200.

[30] "Chiron Announces Promising Data from Clinical Study of Adjuvanted Avian Influenza Vaccine; Results Confirm Previous Clinical Studies: Chiron's MF59 Adjuvant Significantly Enhances Immune Response," Chiron Vaccines, 28 October 2005.

CHAPTER 10: MANDATORY VACCINATION: IS IT POSSIBLE?

[1] Office of the Press Secretary. "President Details Project BioShield," The White House, 3 February 2003. (http://www.whitehouse.gov/news/releases / 2003/02/20030203.html.)

[2] S.1873, "Biodefense and Pandemic Vaccine and Drug Development Act of 2005," The Library of Congress, THOMAS.

[3] "Congress Poised to Rush through Sweeping Immunity for Possibly Unsafe Vaccines and Other Drugs—Americans Likely to Become Human Guinea Pigs," Center for Justice and Democracy, 17 October 2005. (http://www.centerjd.org/free/mythbusters-free/MB_VaccinesAlert.htm.)

[4] "Obey Statement on Defense Appropriations Correction Bill—A Shameful End to a Shameful Congress," United States House of Representatives, 22 December 2005. (http://www.house.gov/appropriations_democrats/press/pr_051222.htm.)

[5] Dodge, Catherine. "Senate Extends Patriot Act, Kills Alaska Drilling." Bloomberg.com 22 December 2005.

[6] "Public Readiness and Emergency Preparedness Act (HR2863)," Advocates for Children's Health Affected by Mercury Poisoning, 17 December 2005. (http://www.a-champ.org/documents/109hr2863_textDIV%22E%22.pdf.)

[7] Office of the Press Secretary. "President Outlines Pandemic Influenza Preparations and Response," The White House, 1 November 2005. (http://www.whitehouse.gov/news/releases/2005/11/20051101-1.html.)

[8] Mello, M. M., Mphil, J. D., PhD, Brennan, T. A. "Legal Concerns and the Influenza Vaccine Shortage," *JAMA* 294 (2005): 1817–1820.

[9] "USC Title 42, Chapter 6A, Subchapter XIX, Part 1: National Vaccine Program," *Cornell Law School*, 2 February 2005.

[10] "National Childhood Vaccine Injury Act Vaccine Injury Table," United States

Department of Health and Human Services.
(http://www.hrsa.gov/osp/vicp/table.htm.)
[11] Kessler, D. A. "Introducing MEDWatch. A new approach to reporting medication and device adverse effects and product problems," *JAMA* 269 (1993): 2765–2768.
[12] "Congress Poised to Rush Through Sweeping Immunity for Possibly Unsafe Vaccines and Other Drugs—Americans Likely to Become Human Guinea Pigs." Center for Justice and Democracy, 17 October 2005.
(http://www.centerjd.org/free/mythbusters-free/MB_VaccinesAlert.htm.)
[13] Statement of the National Vaccine Information Center Co-Founder & President, Barbara Loe Fisher, September 28, 1999, House Oversight Hearing, "Compensating Vaccine Injury: Are Reforms Needed?"
[14] Rusk, Judith. "When it comes to vaccines vs. new drugs, vaccine development loses," *Infectious Diseases in Children*, July 2004.
[15] "FDA Approves New Influenza Vaccine for Upcoming Flu Season," U.S. Food and Drug Administration, 31 August 2005.
(http://www.fda.gov/bbs/topics/news/2005/NEW01227.html.)
[16] "History of Quarantine," The Centers for Disease Control and Prevention, 17 December 2004, National Center For Infectious Diseases Division of Global Migration and Quarantine (formerly the Division of Quarantine).
(http://www.cdc.gov/ncidod/dq/history.htm.)
[17] Office of the Press Secretary. "Executive Order: Amendment to E.O. 13295 Relating to Certain Influenza Viruses and Quarantinable Communicable Diseases," The White House, 1 April 2005.
(http://www.whitehouse.gov/news/releases/ 2005/04/20050401-6.html.)
[18] Misrahi, J. J., Foster, J. A., Shaw, F. E., Cetron, M. S. "HHS/CDC Legal Response to SARS Outbreak," *Emerging Infectious Diseases,* February 2004.
(http://www.cdc.gov/ncidod/EID/vol10no2/03-0721.htm.)
[19] "Public Health Security and Bioterrorism Preparedness and Response Act of 2002," 12 June 2002. PL 107–188. Sec. 142(a)(1).
[20] "Public Health Security and Bioterrorism Preparedness and Response Act of 2002," 12 June 2002. PL 107-188. Sec. 142(b)(2)(B)
[21] Title 42; Chapter 6A, Subchapter II, Part G, § 271 "Penalties for violation of quarantine laws."
[22] Office of the Press Secretary. "Executive Order: Amendment to E.O. 13295 Relating to Certain Influenza Viruses and Quarantinable Communicable Diseases," The White House, 1 April 2005.
(http://www.whitehouse.gov/news/releases/2005/04/20050401-6.html.)
[23] "Dr. Ron Paul Speaks Out on the Real Issue Inherent in Codex," National Health Federation, 3 May 2005. (http://www.thenhf.com/codex_39.htm.)
[24] Jong-wook, Lee, Director General. "Meeting on avian influenza and pandemic human influenza," World Health Organization, 7 November 2005.
(http://www.who.int/dg/lee/speeches/2005/flupandemicgeneva/en/index.html. Last access to this site: February 16, 2006.)
[25] "WHO global influenza preparedness plan," World Health Organization, November 2005. (http://www.who.int/.)

26 McHugh, Josh. "A Chip in Your Shoulder: Should I get an RFID implant?" *Slate Magazine*, 10 November 2004. (http://www.slate.com/id/2109477/. Last accessed February 16, 2006.)

CHAPTER 11: THE SCAM OF TAMIFLU

1 Antiviral Drugs Advisory Committee. "Relenza (Zanamivir for inhalation) GlaxoWelcome Incorporated, for the Treatment of Influenza A and B," Food and Drug Administration, Center for Drug Evaluation and Research, 24 February 1999. (http://www.fda.gov/cder/news/relenza/default.htm.)

2 Ibid., 75–76.

3 Ibid.

4 Ibid.

5 Jolson, Heidi M., MD, MPH. "Relenza® (Zanamivir for inhalation) for treatment of influenza," Food and Drug Administration, Center for Drug Evaluation and Research, 26 October1998.
(http://www.fda.gov/cder/news/relenza/default.htm.)

6 Hayden, F. G. et al. "Use of the selective oral neuraminidase inhibitor oseltamivir to prevent influenza," *New England Journal of Medicine* 341 (1999): 1336–1343.

7 "Canadian Adverse Drug Reaction Newsletter," *Health Canada*, October 2000. (http://www.hc-sc.gc.ca/dhp-mps/alt_formats/hpfb-dgpsa/pdf/medeff/carn-bcei_v10n4_e.pdf.)

8 Antiviral Drugs Advisory Committee. "Relenza (Zanamivir for inhalation) Glaxo Welcome Incorporated, for the Treatment of Influenza A and B." Food and Drug Administration, Center for Drug Evaluation and Research. 24 February 1999. (http://www.fda.gov/cder/news/relenza/default.htm.)

9 Ibid.

10 Hayden, Frederick G. et al. "Use of the Oral Neuraminidase Inhibitor Oseltamivir in Experimental Human Influenza Randomized Controlled Trials for Prevention and Treatment," *JAMA* 282 (1999): 1240–1246.

11 Hayden FG, et al. "Use of the selective oral neuraminidase inhibitor oseltamivir to prevent influenza," *JAMA* 341 (1999): 1336–1343.

12 Associated Press, *Atlanta Journal-Constitution*, 29 November 2004. (http://www.ajc.com/news/content/health/1104/30spray.html.)

13 "Pandemic Influenza Antiviral Stockpile Myth," *Recombinomics*, 23 February 2005. (http://www.recombinomics.com/News/02230505/Antiviral_Myth.html.)

14 QM, Le, et al. "Avian flu: Isolation of drug-resistant H5N1 virus," *Nature* 437 (2005): 1108.

15 Kiso, M., et al. "Resistant influenza A viruses in children treated with oseltamivir: descriptive study," *Lancet* 364 (2004): 759–765. PMID: 15337401.

16 Tamiflu package insert. Food and Drug Administration, Center for Drug Evaluation and Research, 24 July 2001.
(http://www.fda.gov/cder/foi/label/2001/21246s3lbl.pdf.)

17 "East Asia: No new evidence of Tamiflu-resistant H5N1," University of Washington, 7 October 2005.

(http://depts.washington.edu/einet/?a=printArticle&print=907.)

18 "BPCA Executive Summary. NDA 21-087/NDA 21–246 Tamiflu capsules and for oral suspension," Food and Drug Administration, Center for Drug Evaluation and Research, 28 June 2004.
(http://www.fda.gov/cder/foi/esum/2004/21087,21246_ Tamiflu_ clinical_ BPCA.pdf.)

19 "Tamiflu™ Granted FDA Approval for Treatment of Flu in Children," Roche Pharmaceuticals, 14 December 2000. (http://www.rocheusa.com/newsroom/ current/2000/pr2000121401.html.)

20 "BPCA Executive Summary. NDA 21-087/NDA 21-246 Tamiflu capsules and for oral suspension," Food and Drug Administration, Center for Drug Evaluation and Research, 28 June 2004. (http://www.fda.gov/cder/foi/esum /2004/21087,21246_Tamiflu _clinical_BPCA.pdf.)

21 "DIMACS Working Group on Adverse Event/Disease Reporting, Surveillance, and Analysis," Rutgers University 16–18 (October 2002).
(http://dimacs.rutgers.edu/Workshops/AdverseEvent/announcement.html.)

22 Department of Health and Human Services, Public Health Service, Food and Drug Administration, Center for Drug Evaluation and Research Memorandum, Food and Drug Administration, 25 August 2005.

23 Department of Health and Human Services, Public Health Service, Food and Drug Administration, Center for Drug Evaluation and Research Memorandum, Food and Drug Administration, 25 August 2005. PID# D040223.

24 "Rumsfeld Garners $1 Million In Recent Run-Up Of Gilead Stock Report," *The Morningstar Report*, 2 November 2005.

25 "Richard Cheney Files," Gerald R. Ford Library, White House Operations. 1974–77.
(http://www.ford.utexas.edu/library/guides/Finding%20Aids/Cheney,%20Rich ard%20-%20Files.htm.)

26 Felsenthal, Carol. "Donald Rumsfeld's biography: The Don," *Chicago Magazine*, June 2001.

27 Dewey, David Lawrence. "$350 Million Plus Lawsuit Filed Against Nutrasweet Monsanto Aspartame Sweetener," *Dewey's World*, 15 September 2004.
(http://www.dldewey.com/rico.htm.)

28 (For more on the timeline of aspartame NutraSweet®, see Rense.com at http://www.rense.com/general33/legal.htm.)

29 Ibid.

30 Turner, James S. "Donald Rumsfeld and the Aspartame NutraSweet Fiasco," *Namaste Magazine*.
(http://www.namastepublishing.co.uk/Aspartame%20Fiasco.htm.)

31 LeDuc, James W., Damon, Inger, Meegan, James M., Relman, David A., Huggins, John, Jahrling, Peter B. "Smallpox Research Activities: U.S.Interagency Collaboration, 2001," *Emerging Infectious Diseases*, 8 (2002).

32 Elias Paul. "Roche promises new plant for bird flu drug."*The Boston Globe*, 18 Oct. 2005. The Associated Press.

CHAPTER 12: HOW THE CURRENT HYPE BEGAN

1 Ku, A. S. and Chan, L. T. "The first case of H5N1 avian influenza infection in a human with complications of adult respiratory distress syndrome and Reye's syndrome," *Journal of Paediatrics and Child Health*, 35(2) (April 1999): 207–209.

2 "Influenza A(H5N1) widespread in Hong Kong market," *Infectious Disease News*, March 1998. (http://www. Infectiousdiseasenews.com.)

CHAPTER 13: THE KILLING FIELDS

1 "Avian influenza update 31," World Health Organization, 22 September 2005.

2 FAOstat. Statistical database of Food and Agriculture Organization of the United Nations, Rome Italy. FAO. (1998).

3 All information regarding raising domestic chickens and ducks in Southeast Asia was obtained from the Web site for the International Network for Family Poultry Development. (http://www.fao.org/ag/againfo/subjects/en/infpd/home.html.)

4 "Avian influenza update 31," World Health Organization, 22 September 2005.

5 Cheng, Tony "Thai poultry farmers grieve losses," BBC News, 27 January 2004. (http://news.bbc.co.uk/1/hi/world/asia-pacific/3430593.stm.)

6 "Avian Influenza–Death Toll: 50 Million and Rising," Sec. 4: Killing Methods. *United Poultry Concerns*, 12 February 2004. (http://www.upc-online.org/ health/21304flu.htm. Web site last accessed February 17, 2006.)

7 "Turkey, Romania slaughter more fowl to combat bird flu," Channel News Asia. 12 October 2005.

8 "Thai Animal Activist Says Chicken Cull Inhumane," Channel News Asia, 30 January 2004. Agence France Presse. (http://www.channelnewsasia.com/.)

9 "U.S. Egg Industry." United Egg Producers. U.S. Dept. of Agriculture, American Egg Board, USAPEEC. (http://www.unitedegg.org/useggindustry_generalstats.aspx.)

10 Franklin, Col. Steve, Erickson, Debbie, Bozzard, Jim, and Shorter, Byron. "2003 Agribusiness Group Paper," National Defense University.

11 "The Modern Chicken Industry: Suffering for Humanity," Vassar College Department of Geology & Geography. (http://geologyandgeography.vassar.edu/projects/saed/Chicken Pulin.htm#_ftn6.)

12 Davis, Karen PhD "The Battery Hen: Her Life Is Not For The Birds."

13 (For more information on this horrifying industry and what you can do, contact United Poultry Concerns at: www.upc-online.org)

14 "Safety in the Meat and Poultry Industry, while Improving, Could Be Further Strengthened," Government Accountability Office, January 2005. (http://www.gao.gov/new.items/d0596.pdf.)

15 "Top 10 Broiler Companies," U.S. Poultry & Egg Association, 2 February 2005. (http://www.poultryegg.org/EconomicInfo/.)

16 Ireland, Doug. "Birds of a Feather," *City Pages*, 7 January 1998. (http://www.city-pages.com/databank/19/892/article4074.asp.)

[17] "Blood, Sweat, and Fear Workers' Rights in U.S. Meat and Poultry Plants." *Human Rights Watch.* January 2005.
(http://www.hrw.org/reports/2005/usa0105/usa0105.pdf.)
[18] Ransom, Steven. "Without Bars," La Leva di Archimede Association for freedom of choice. (http://www.laleva.cc/food/withoutbars.html.)
[19] Delforge, Isabelle. "Thailand: the world's kitchen," *Le Monde diplomatique*, 7 July 2004. (http://mondediplo.com/2004/07/05thailand.)
[20] Ibid.
[21] "Playing Chicken Thaksin Shinawatra's government comes clean on the extent of avian flu in Thailand," *TIME Asia.* 2 February 2004. (http://www.time.com/.)
[22] Ibid.
[23] Delforge, Isabelle. "The Politics of The Bird Flu in Thailand," *Focus on the Global South*, 19 April 2004. (http://www.focusweb.org/ content/view/273/29/.)
[24] "Ha Tay wages grueling war on avian flu," *Viet Nam News*, 5 February 2004. (http://vietnamnews.vnagency.com.vn/2004-02/04/Stories/02.htm. Last accessed February 17, 2006.)
[25] Ibid.
[26] Delforge, Isabelle. "The flu that made agribusiness stronger," *Focus on the Global South*, 5 July 2004. (http://www.focusweb.org/content/view/363/28/.)
[27] Cheng, Tony. "Thai poultry farmers grieve losses." BBC News. 27 January 2004. (http://news.bbc.co.uk/1/hi/world/asia-pacific/3430593.stm. Accessed February 17, 2006.)
[28] Delforge, "The flu that made agribusiness stronger."
[29] Ibid.
[30] Ibid.
[31] "Ho Chi Minh City to slaughter all poultry because of bird flu," *AsiaNews*, 17 February 2005
(http://www.asianews.it/view.php?l=en&art=2592.)
[32] Minh Ho Binh. "Vietnam cities hasten mass poultry slaughter," Reuters, 15 November 2005.
http://www.redorbit.com/news/international/305878/vietnam_cities_hasten_mass_poultry_slaughter/
[33] Bong, Ba Bui, MD. "Measures to Control Avian Influenza and Pandemic Preparedness in Vietnam," World Health Organization, 7–9 November 2005. (http://www.who.int/mediacentre/events/2005/05_Vietnam_Bui_Ba_Bong_L.pdf.)
[34] Brahmbhatt, Milan. "Avian and Human Pandemic Influenza – Economic and Social Impacts," World Health Organization, 7–9 November 2005.
[35] Foster, Sarah. "Police State, U.K. 'You're not killing my animals!' Refuge owner battles UK government over slaughter policy," *WorldNetDaily*, 27 April 2002.
[36] Ibid.
[37] "Tyson Foods Victorious in IBP Bidding War Now Nation's No.1 Beef, Poultry Processor," Mindfully.org, 11 January 2001.
(http://www.mindfully.org/Industry/Tyson-Foods-Victorious-IBP.htm.)
[38] Ibid.
[39] Ransom, Steven. "Without Bars," La Leva di Archimede Association for freedom

of choice.
(http://www.laleva.cc/food/withoutbars.html.)
[40] Farah, Joseph. "Who wins in China's chicken war?" *World Net Daily*, 31 December 1997. (http://www.wnd.com/ news/article. asp? ARTICLE_ID=14399.)
[41] Fan, Yi. "Old Trade, New Opportunities," *China Today,* August 2005.
[42] "China's 100 Richest Business People," *Forbes.* 12 November 2001. (http://www.forbes.com/global/2001/1112/032.html. Accessed February 17, 2006.)
[43] Flannery, Russell ed. "China's 40 Richest," *Forbes,* 3 November 2005. (http://www.forbes.com/2005/11/01/china-richest-list_05china_land.html. Accessed February 17, 2006.)
[44] Flannery, Russell. "Not Just Chicken Feed," *Forbes,* 14 November 2005. (http://www.forbes.com/business/global/2005/1114/075A.html.
[45] "Virus outbreaks may change poultry raising." *China Daily.* Agence France-Presse. 1 December 2005. (http://www.chinadaily.com.cn/english/doc/2005-12/01/content_499324.htm. Accessed February 17, 2006.) Accessed February 17, 2006.)
[46] Yong, Wu and Na, He. "Bird flu hits egg farmers," *China Daily,* 15 November 2005.(http://www.chinadaily.com.cn/english/doc/2005-11/15/content_494691.htm.)
[47] "Mass slaughter of fowl in India after bird flu outbreak reported. *International Herald Tribune,* 19 February 2006.
http://www.iht.com/bin/print_ipub.php?file=/ articles/2006/02/19/news/web.0219flu.php

CHAPTER 14: SICK CHICKS IN THE U.S.

[1] "H7 Avian flu found in Maryland, 4th State with the Virus," *Bloomberg*, 7 March 2005. (http://quote.bloomberg.com.)
[2] "Compassion over Killing (COK) Report: Animal Suffering in the Broiler Industry," *Compassion over Killing.* (http://www.cok.net/images/pdf/COKBroilerReport.pdf.)
[3] Davis, Karen PhD "Re: Humane Treatment of Domestic Livestock," *United Poultry Concerns,* 27 June 2003. (http://www.njfarms.org/UPC.pdf.)
[4] Bagel, Ann. "Excess ammonia levels killed Tyson chickens," Meetingplace.com, 5 April 2004.
[5] Runkle, Nathan. "Covert Investigation Exposes Cruelty at Ohio's Largest Egg Farms," *Egg Cruelty,* 17 October 2001. (http://www.eggcruelty.com/covert_investigation_press_release.asp.)
[6] Hayes, Rich. "Antibiotics Overused in Chickens," Common Dreams News Center, 23 July 2001. *The Baltimore Sun.* (http://www.commondreams.org/views01/0723-04.htm.)
[7] Davis, Karen PhD, "Re: Humane Treatment of Domestic Livestock."
[8] Smyth, J. R., Erf, G. F., Sreekumar, G. P.: "Do viruses and/or growing environment affect the expression of vitilego in Smyth line chickens?" *Pigment Cell Research,* 10

(1997): 108.

9 Sreekumar, G. P., Smyth, J. R., Jr., Ambady, S., Ponce de Leon, F. A. "Analysis of the effect of endogenous viral genes in the Smyth line chicken model for autoimmune vitilego," *American Journal of Pathology*, 156 (2000): 1099-1107. PMID: 10702426 (http://ajp.amjpathol.org/cgi/content/full/156/3/1099.)

10 University of Arkansas Division of Agriculture report.

11 Andrews, Andy. "Chicks Become 'Superbirds' If Critical Needs are Met," *Lancaster Farming*, A1 28 March 1992.

12 "Birds Exploited for Meat," Poultry.Org.
(http://www.poultry.org/suffering.htm.)

13 Davis, Karen PhD, "The Battery Hen: Her Life Is Not For The Birds."

14 "Picower researcher's transgenic technique could lead to avian flu-resistant birds," Massachusetts Institute of Technology. (http://web.mit.edu/newsoffice/2005/birds.html.)

15 Henderson, Mark. "Scientists aim to beat flu with genetically modified chickens," *The London Times*, October 29, 2005. (http://www.timesonline.co.uk/article/0,,25149-1847760,00.html.)

16 Lean, Geoffrey. "GM Industry Puts Human Gene into Rice," Common Dreams News Center, 24 April 2005. *The Independent* (United Kingdom).
(http://www.commondreams.org/headlines05/0424-06.htm.)

17 "StarLink fiasco wreaks havoc in the heartland Developer wants EPA to approve seed for food supply," The Campaign to Label Genetically Engineered Foods, *USA Today*, 27 October 2000.
(http://thecampaign.org/newsupdates/oct00dd.htm. Accessed February 17, 2006.)

18 "Top Chinese agribusiness predicts importation of corn," AgLines, 9 September 2005.

19 "Terminator Technology: Suicide Seeds Are Back!" Ban Terminator. July 2005. (http//www.**banterminator**.org/content/download/275/2646/file/Terminator%20background.pdf. Accessed February 17, 2006.)

20 Wan, Ho Mae and Burcher, Sam. "Cows Ate GM Maize & Died," The Institute of Science in Society, 13 January 2004. (http://www.i-sis.org.uk/CAGMMAD.php.)

21 Montague Peter. "The Global Spread of GMO Crops," *Counter Punch*. 7–8 January 2006

CHAPTER 15: SICK MIGRATORY BIRDS: CANARIES IN THE COAL MINES

1 Miguel, Edward and Roland, Gérard. "The Long Run Impact of Bombing Vietnam," Department of Economics, University of California, Berkeley, October 2005. (http://emlab.berkeley.edu/users/emiguel/miguel_vietnam.pdf.)

2 Green, Gerard. "Agent Blue and the Business of Killing Rice," *Focus on the Global South*, 3 June 2004.

3 DiGangi, Joseph and Petrlik, Jindrich. "The Egg Report," *Oztoxics*, April, 2005.

4 Westing, Arthur H. *Herbicides in War: Long-term Ecological and Human Consequences*, London: Taylor & Francis, 1984.

5 Dwernychuk, L. W., Cau, H. D., Hatfield C. T., Boivin T. G., Hung, T.M., Dung, P. T., Thai, N. D. "Dioxin reservoirs in southern Viet Nam—a legacy of Agent Orange," *Chemosphere* 47 (2002): 117-137. PMID: 11993628.
6 "Contaminated Sediment in Water," U.S. Environmental Protection Agency. (http://www.epa.gov/waterscience/cs/aboutcs/sources.html.)
7 "Greenpeace: EPA Review of Dioxins Underestimates Chemicals' Sources," *The Sludge Newsletter*, August 1994.
8 "How Toxic is Your Diet?" *Inter Press Services*, 20 November 1997. (http://www.ejnet.org/dioxin/diet.html.)
9 Quynh, Hoang Trong, MD, et al. "Long-term consequences of Vietnam War," *Nordic News Network*, Report to the Environmental Conference on Cambodia, Laos and Vietnam. (http://www.nnn.se/vietnam/health.pdf.)
10 "Greenpeace: EPA Review of Dioxins Underestimates Chemicals' Sources," *The Sludge Newsletter*, August 1994.
11 Schecter, A., Quynh, H. T., Pavuk, M., Papke, O., Malisch, R., Constable, J. D. "Food as a source of dioxin exposure in the residents of Bien Hoa City, Vietnam," *Journal of Occupational and Environmental Medicine* 45 (2003): 781–788. PMID: 12915779.
12 Warren, T. K., Mitchell, K. A., Lawrence, B. P. "Exposure to 2,3,7,8-Tetrachlorodibenzo-p-dioxin (TCDD) Suppresses the Humoral and Cell-Mediated Immune Responses to Influenza A Virus without Affecting Cytolytic Activity in the Lung," *Toxicological Sciences* 56 (2000): 114–,123.
13 Burleson, G. R., et al. "Effect of 2,3,7,8-tetrachlorodibenzo-p-dioxin (TCDD) on influenza virus host resistance in mice," *Toxicological Sciences*, 29 (1996): 40–47.
14 Warren, T. K., Mitchell, K. A., Lawrence, B. P. "Exposure to 2,3,7,8-Tetrachlorodibenzo-p-dioxin (TCDD) Suppresses the Humoral and Cell-Mediated Immune Responses to Influenza A Virus without Affecting Cytolytic Activity in the Lung," *Toxicological Sciences* 56 (2000): 114–123.
15 Luebke, R. W, et al. "Mortality in dioxin-exposed mice infected with influenza: mitochondrial toxicity (Reye's-like syndrome) versus enhanced inflammation as the mode of action," *Toxicological Sciences* 69 (2002): 109–116.
16 Chan, M. C., et al. "Proinflammatory cytokine responses induced by influenza A(H5N1) viruses in primary human alveolar and bronchial epithelial cells," *Respiratory Research* 6 (2005): 135. PMID 16283933.
17 Yungandagencies, Chester. "Bird flu risk to young revealed by experts," *The Standard* (Hong Kong), 12 November 2005. (http://www.thestandard.com/hk/news.)
18 Cooke, Marcus, Clark, George C., Goeyens, Leo, Baeyens, Willy. "Environmental Bioanalysis of Dioxin," *Today's Chemist* 9 (2000): 15–19.
19 "Photos of 1000's of Bird Flu Deaths on Bird Island Qinghai China," *Recombinomics*, 3 June 2005
20 "Nuclear Waste and Weapons on the Tibetan Plateau," *International Campaign for Tibet*. (http://www.savetibet.org/news/ positionpapers / nuclearwaste.php.)
21 Ibid.
22 "Tibet: Environment and Development Issues," *Tibet Environmental Watch*,

Chapter 7: Nuclear Threats, 27 April 2000.
(http://www.tew.org/tibet2000/t2.ch7.nuclear.html.)
23 "Radionuclides in the Columbia River," Washington State Department of
Health, Hanford Health Information Network.
(http://www.doh.wa.gov/Hanford/publications/overview/columbia.html.)
24 Markham, O. D., Halford, D. K., Rope, S. K., Kuzo, G. B. "Plutonium, Am, Cm
and Sr in ducks maintained on radioactive leaching ponds in Southeastern Idaho,"
Health Physics 55 (1988): 517–524.
25 Sumit, K Sen. "Avian Influenza (or Bird Flu) and India," *The Birds of Kolkata*.
(http://www.kolkatabirds.com/birdflu.htm.)
26 "Asia-Pacific Migratory Waterbird Conservation Strategy: 1996–2000,"
Australian Government Department of the Environment and Heritage
(1996–2000). Wetlands International–Asia Pacific.
27 Orent, Wendy. "Sure, it kills birds, but it won't kill you," *Los Angeles Times*, 23
October 2005.
28 Dyer, Gwynne. "Bird flu panic not misplaced," *The Winnipeg Free Press*, 17
October 2005.
29 "Avian influenza A(H5N1)–update 31: Situation (poultry) in Asia: need for a
long-term response, comparison with previous outbreaks," World Health
Organization, 2 March 2004. (http://www.who.int.)
30 Rosenthal, Elisabeth. Migrating Birds Didn't Carry Flu. *New York Times*.
May 11, 2006   http://www.nytimes.com
31 "Scientists hunt for deadly bird flu in Alaska," *Associated Press*, 22 May 2006.
32 "State To Test Wild Birds For Avian Flu," *Associated Press*, 13 June 2006.
33 Weigand, Polly. "The Use of U.S. Pesticides in the Tropical Americas," St.
Lawrence University (1998).
34 "Avian influenza A(H5N1)–update 31: Situation (poultry) in Asia: need for a
long-term response, comparison with previous outbreaks," World Health
Organization, 2 March 2004. (http://www.who.int/csr/don/2004_03_02/en/.)

Chapter 16: Sick Humans

1 "Avian Influenza A(H5N1) Infection in Humans." *New England Journal of
Medicine* 353 (2005): 1374–1385.
2 Krukowski, John, "Cracking Dioxin's Secrets," *Special Report–Pollution
Engineering*, 15 January 1992. (http://www.biosolids.org/docs/dioxin.pdf.)
3 Olden, Kenneth PhD "TCDD–Dioxin—is Listed as 'Known Human Carcinogen'
in Federal Government's Ninth Report On Carcinogens." National Institute of
Environmental Health Sciences, 19 January 2001.
(http://www.niehs.nih.gov/oc/news/dioxadd.htm.)
4 "Vietnam Veterans and Agent Orange Exposure." United States Department of
Veterans Affairs Employee Education System, March 2002.
5 Grassman, Jean A., Masten, Scott A., Walker, Nigel J., Lucier, George W.
"Animal Models of Human Response to Dioxins," *Environmental Health Perspectives*
106 (1998).

6 Stellman, J. M., Stellman, S. D., Christian, R., Weber, T., Tomasallo, C. "The extent and patterns of usage of Agent Orange and other herbicides in Vietnam," *Nature* 422 (2003): 681–7. PMID: 12700752.

7 Quynh, Hoang Trong MD, et al. "Long-term consequences of Vietnam War," Nordic News Network's Report to the Environmental Conference on Cambodia, Laos, and, Vietnam. (http://www.nnn.se/vietnam/health.pdf.)

8 Schecter, A. J., et al. "Pesticide application and increased dioxin body burden in male and female agricultural workers in China," *Journal of Occupational and Environmental Medicine* 38 (1996): 906–911.

9 Schecter A., et al. "Food as a source of dioxin exposure in the residents of Bien Hoa City, Vietnam," *Journal of Occupational and Environmental Medicine* 45 (2003): 781–788. PMID: 12915779.

10 Schecter, A, et al. "Dioxin, dibenzofuran, and polychlorinated biphenyl (PCB) levels in food from Agent Orange-sprayed and non-sprayed areas of Laos," *Journal of Toxicology and Environmental Health* 66 (2003): 2165–2186. PMID: 14710598.

11 "Contamination of Chicken Eggs from Barangay Aguado in Philippines by Dioxins, PCBs and Hexachlorobenzene," Global Alliance for Incinerator Alternatives/Global Anti-Incinerator Alliance, 21 April 2005.

12 DiGangi, Joseph and Petrlik, Jindrich. "The Egg Report," *Oztoxics*, April 2005. (http://www.oztoxics.org /ipepweb/egg/egg%20reports/GLOBAL_eggsreport %20FINAL.pdf.)

13 Petreas, M. X., et al. "Biotransfer and bioaccumulation of PCDD/PCDFs from soil: controlled exposure studies of chickens," *Chemosphere* 23(1991): 1731–1741.

14 "Evaluation of Dioxins in Crab and Geoduck Tissue From a Lower Elwha Klallam Tribe Fishing Area Near Port Angeles, Washington," Agency for Toxic Substance and Disease Registry ATSDR, 28 February 2005. (http://www.atsdr.cdc.gov/HAC/PHA/RayonierMill022805-WA/RayonierMills022805-WA.pdf.)

15 "Executive Summary: Assessment of the health risk of dioxins: re-evaluation of the Tolerable Daily Intake (TDI)," World Health Organization, 25–29 May 1998.)

16 "China egg production gets into full swing," *AP-Food Technology*, 7 February 2005. (http://ap-foodtechnology.com/news/ng.asp?id=53273&n=wh27&ec=%23 emailcode.)

17 Dooley, Erin E. "Reviving China's Ruined Rivers," *Environmental Health Perspectives* 110 (2002).

18 Nierenberg, Danielle. "Industrial Animal Agriculture—the next global health crisis?" World Society for the Protection of Animals, November 2004.

19 Schmidt, Charles W. "Economy and Environment: China Seeks a Balance," *Environmental Health Perspectives* 110 (2002).

20 Table: Changhua, Wu, et al. "Water Pollution and Human Health in China," *Environmental Health Perspectives* 107 (1999).

21 O'Neill, Marie S, et al. "Health, Wealth, and Air Pollution: Advancing Theory and Methods," *Environmental Health Perspectives* 111 (2003).

22 Schmidt, Charles W. "Economy and Environment: China Seeks a Balance," *Environmental Health Perspectives* 110 (2002).

23 "Bird Flu Spreads, 11 Cities Quarantined," *Zaman Daily Newspaper*, 8 January 2006. (http://www.zaman.com/?bl=national&alt= &trh=20060108&hn=28404.)
24 Ozler, Murat H. "Active Saltwater Encroachment (from Lake Van) in the Van Aquifer, East Turkey," The University of Mississippi. First International Conference on Saltwater Intrusion and Coastal Aquifers—Monitoring, Modeling, and Management. Essaouira, Morocco 23–25 April 2001.
(http://www.olemiss.edu/sciencenet/saltnet/swica1/Ozler.pdf.)
25 (Information on conditions in Armenia and throughout the Southern Caucasus obtained from, "Chapter 2. State of the Caucasus Environment and Policy Measures: a retrospective from 1972 to 2002," *Caucasus Environment Outlook*, 2002. (http://www.grid.unep.ch/product/publication/CEO-for-Internet/CEO/ch2_4_3.htm.)
26 Hewing, Amy. "Water Quality and Public Health Monitoring of Surface Waters in the Kura-Araks River Basin of Armenia, Azerbaijan, and Georgia." The University of New Mexico, July 2003. (http://www.unm.edu/~wrp/wrp-8.pdf.)
27 Gasparian, Anahit. "Nuclear Power Plant In an Earthquake Zone," ISAR Resources For Environmental Activists.
(http://www.isar.org/pubs/ST/ARmedzamor48.html.)
28 "Armenia: nuclear power plant will restart," *News From Russia*, 17 November 2005. (http://newsfromrussia.com/world/2005/11/17/67913.html.)
29 Bahar, Tahsin, MD. "JRC Information Events in Turkey Chemicals and Chemical Industry," EU Sixth Framework Programme (FP6) National Coordination Office (NCO), 18 October 2005.
(http://www.fp6.org.tr/web/ETKINLIKLER/Bilim_Aras_Gunleri/Bahar.pdf.)
30 "Chemicals," D?? Ekonomik ?li?kiler Kurulu Foreign Economic Relations Board, June 2002.
http://www.deik.org.tr/bultenler/2003320154121sectors-chemicals-june02.pdf.)
31 "Contamination of chicken eggs near the Koshice municipal waste incinerator in Slovakia by dioxins, PCBs and hexachlorobenzene," *Oztoxics*, 16 March 2005. International POPs Elimination Network (IPEN). (http://www.oztoxics.org/ipep-web/egg/HotspotReports/Slovakia_eggsreport.pdf.)
32 Eaton, Janet PhD "Ecological and Health Consequences of the NATO Bombings of Pancevo and other Petrochemical and Chemical Industrial Complexes," International Action Center, 10 June 2000.
33 Al-Azzawi, Dr. Souad N. "Testimony on Radioactive Contamination in Iraq Environmental Damages of Military Operations During the Invasion of Iraq (IIMO) (2003–2005)." World Tribunal on Iraq, 25 June 2005.
34 Johnson, Larry. "Iraqi cancers, birth defects blamed on U.S. depleted uranium," *Seattle Post-Intelligencer*, 12 November 2002.
35 Edwards, Rob. "WHO 'suppressed' scientific study into depleted uranium cancer fears in Iraq," *Sunday Herald* (Glasgow), 22 February 2004.
36 Nebehay, Stephanie. "UN's WHO confirms bird flu killed Iraqi girl," Reuters, 2 February 2006.

Chapter 17: Tying It All Together

1 DeAngelo, LeAnna. *Germs On Our Mind: The Psychology of Contagion*, Washington: New Academia, 2005.

2 Margulis, Lyn PhD "Germs and Viruses," Soil And Health Library, 1980. (http://www.soilandhealth.org/02/0201hyglibcat/020122horne.21stcentury/020122ch5.html.)

3 Hamowy, Ronald. "The Early Development of Medical Licensing Laws in the United States, 1875–1900," Ludwig von Mises Institute, Department of History, University of Alberta. (http://www.mises.org/journals/jls/3_1/3_1_5.pdf.)

4 Chikly, Bruno J. D.O. "Manual Techniques Addressing the Lymphatic System: Origins and Development," *The Journal of the American Osteopathic Association* 105 (2005): 457–464.

5 Avian Flu "Endemic" in Southeast Asia, and "Inevitable" in Europe," PRNewswire, 5 January 2006. (http://www.prnewswire.co.uk/cgi/news/release?id=161348.)

6 "Toxic Ignorance," *Environmental Defense*, 1997. (http://edf.org/documents/ 243_toxicignorance.pdf.)

7 "Generations X Results WWF's European Family Biomonitoring Survey," *World Wide Fund for Nature*, 2005. (http://assets.panda. org/downloads /generationsx-summary.pdf.)

8 "Trade Secrets: A Moyers Report," Public Broadcasting Service, 2001. (http://www.pbs.org/tradesecrets.)

9 "Bill Moyers' test results," Public Broadcasting Service. (http://www.pbs.org/tradesecrets /problem/popup_bb_02.html.)

10 Ibid.

11 "Body Burden—The Pollution in Newborns," Environmental Working Group, 14 July 2005. (http://www.ewg.org/reports/bodyburden2/execsumm.php.)

12 Khamchoo, Wattana. "IMMIGRANTS: Thousands given Thai nationality," *The Nation*, 3 January 2006. (http://www.nationmultimedia.com/.)

13 "Financial crisis hits Bangladesh poultry sector," Onlypunjab.com, 19 February 2005. (http://onlypunjab.com/fullstory2k5-insight—status-22-newsID-12184.html.)

14 Alam, Julhas. "Bangladesh takes steps to prevent bird flu outbreak," Associated Press, 27 November 2005. (http://news.inq7.net/breaking/index.php?index=3&story_id=57932.)

15 Oboh, Mike. "Bird flu reaches Africa, kills Nigerian poultry," Reuters, 8 February 2006. (http://www.alertnet.org/thenews/newsdesk/L08253227.htm.)

16 Curtis, Clifton. "Time to clean up the chemicals in Africa," *Khaleej Times*, 6 February 2006.

17 "Pulp Mill Devastates Swans' Sanctuary In Chile," *World Wildlife Fund*, 21 November 2005.

18 Kumar, Lalit. "Mercury may have caused bird deaths," *The Times of India*, 6 February 2006.

19 Schecter, A., et al. "Food as a source of dioxin exposure in the residents of Bien

Hoa City, Vietnam," *Journal of Occupational and Environmental Medicine* 45 (2003): 781–800.

[20] "The American People's Dioxin Report," Center for Health Environment and Justice, 13 April 1999.)

[21] "Dioxins in Total Diet Survey 2001 Samples: Your Questions Answered," Food Standards Agency.
(http://www.foodstandards.gov.uk/multimedia/ faq/ dioxins _ qanda/.)

[22] "Cancer Risk; Re-analysis of data finds no evidence of dioxin cancer threshold," Environmental Justice, *Cancer Weekly*, 23 October 2003.
(http://www.ejnet.org/dioxin/nosafedose.html.)

[23] Changhua, Wu, et al. "Water Pollution and Human Health in China," *Environmental Health Perspectives* 107 (1999).

[24] Schecter, A., Pavuk, M., Papke, O., Ryan, J. J. "Dioxin, dibenzofuran, and coplanar PCB levels in Laotian blood and milk from agent orange-sprayed and nonsprayed areas, 2001," *Journal of Toxicology and Environmental Health* 66 (2003): 2067–2075.

[25] "Workshop Report on the Application of 2,3,7,8-TCDD Toxicity Equivalence Factors to Fish and Wildlife," U.S. Environmental Protection Agency, Risk Assessment Forum, August 2001.

[26] Higgens, Marguerite. "Poultry Problems," *The Washington Times*, 13 March 2004.

[27] Grassman, Jean A., Masten, Scott A., Walker, Nigel J., Lucier, George W. "Animal Models of Human Response to Dioxins," *Environmental Health Perspectives* 106 (1998)

[28] Heller, Charles E. MAJ(P) USAR. "Chemical Warfare in World War I The American Experience, 1917–1918." US Army Command and General Staff College. September 1984, Combat Studies Institute. (http://www-cgsc.army.mil/carl/ resources/csi/Heller/HELLER.asp.)

[29] Redican, Lindsay. "The Forgotten Killer," Haverford College.
(http://www.haverford.edu/biology /edwards /disease/viral_essays/redican-virus.htm.)

[30] Kolata, Gina. FLU: The Story of the Great Influenza Pandemic of 1918 and the Search for the Virus That Caused It, Farrar, Straus, and Giroux, 1999.

[31] "History of Epidemics and Plagues," University of Hartford, October 2001.

[32] Sparks, S. & Self. S., et al. "Super-eruptions: global effects and future threats," The Geological Society of London, June 2005.

CHAPTER 18: GETTING INVOLVED: THE ACTIVIST'S PLAY BOOK

[1] Ching, Li Lim. "GM Crops Increase Pesticide Use," Institute of Science in Society, 12 November 2003.

[2] Landes, Lynn. Pharmaceuticals, Pesticides, and Radiation Cause Breast Cancer . . . While Wealthy Non-Profits and Feds Protect Industry, Common Dreams News Center, 23 October 2002.

[3] "Acetochlor." Cornell University Pesticide Management Education Program, June 1996. (http://pmep.cce.cornell.edu/profiles/extoxnet/24d-captan/ acetochlor-ext.html.)

[4] "Weed Killers by the Glass Health Effects of Herbicides," Environmental

Working Group. (http://www.ewg.org/reports/Weed_Killer/weed1.html.)

5 Novartis Oncology. At Novartis Oncology our approach is simple. We call it 'Think. Do.'?"
(http://www.us.novartisoncology.com/info/about/index.jsp?checked=y.)

6 "Tamoxifen: Questions and Answers," National Cancer Institute.
(http://www.cancer.gov/cancertopics/factsheet/Therapy/tamoxifen.)

7 Herper, Matthew. "Crops, Shmops. Pharmacia Spins Off Monsanto," *Forbes*, 28 November 2001. (http://www.forbes.com.)

8 Smith Jeffery M. *Seeds of Deception*, Fairfield: Yes! Books, 2003.

9 Weiss Rick. "Biotech Food Raises a Crop of Questions,"*The Washington Post*, A1, 15 August, 1999.

10 A good place to start is with the book by Dr. Sherry Rogers, *Detoxify or Die*, published in 2002.

INDEX

A

ACIP (Advisory Committee of Immun. Practices) 113, 251
Adjuvant formula 94
Adjuvants 93-96, 98-101, 269
   oil-based 95
   squalene-based 97, 99
   squalene-containing 100
Aerosolized saline 129
AERS (Adverse Event Reporting System) 133
Africa 43, 194, 229, 248, 281
Agent Blue 181, 276
Agent Orange 179-183, 198-201, 203, 206, 207, 232, 245, 277, 279
Agent Pink 181
Agribusinesses 148, 149, 156-158, 165, 168, 242, 243, 247, 248, 274
AhR-dioxin 188
Alaska 194, 278
Aluminum 99, 101
   hydroxide 95
   phosphate 95
   sulfate 95
American Legion Convention 35
Ammonia 169, 170, 216
Anaphylaxis 95, 97, 111, 112
Ankara, Turkey 215
Antibodies
   protective 46
   vaccine-induced 46
Antibody response 71, 86, 93, 96, 99
Antigenic drifts 20, 121, 131
Antigens 14, 19, 27, 70, 72, 86, 87, 90, 93, 122, 127, 255, 258
Antiviral drugs 105, 122, 129
Aquifer, underground 213
Aras River 280
Armenia 212-214, 280

Artificial sweetener 136
Aspartame 136-138, 228
AstraZeneca 160, 244
Australia 3, 18, 97, 229
Autoimmune
   arthritis 95, 97
   disorders 95, 243
   vaccine-induced 171
   vitilego 276
Aviagen 154, 166, 172, 178
Avian
   erythroblastosis virus 77
   influenza
      update 273
      viruses 19, 168, 194
   myeloblastosis virus 77
   myelocytoma virus 77
Azerbaijan 212, 280

B

Babies, 23-month-old 82
Baculovirus 90
Bangladesh 228, 229, 281
Baverstock, Keith 218
Bien Hoa City 199, 200
Biological products 69, 108, 134, 251, 253, 254
Bioterrorism Act of 2002 115, 116
Bird Island 188, 190, 191
Bovine
   sera 79
   viruses 80
   BSE, Bovine Spongiform
Encephalopathy 92
Breast cancer 244
Burma 200, 229
Bush administration 109, 161

C

Cambodia 143, 182, 200, 201, 211, 228, 277, 279
Canadian Adverse Drug Reaction

Laos 143, 182, 200, 201, 211, 232, 277, 279
Lawsuits, vaccine injury 33
Leavenworth Papers 235, 239
Legionnaire's Disease 35
Lewandowsky, Stephen 3, 4, 261
Liaoning Province 165, 210, 231
Liu Yongxing 163, 164, 174
Lobbyists 66, 106, 249
Low-pathogenic influenza viruses 197

M
Malaysia 148
Mandatory vaccination 103, 105, 107, 109, 111, 113-115, 117, 119, 120, 245, 269
Marek's Disease 171
Masks 236, 238
Mass vaccination 2, 29, 32, 33, 36, 44, 63, 73, 117, 119, 120
  mandatory 41, 103
Matsumoto,Gary 96, 99, 268
McReardon, Benjamin 80
MDCK, Madin-Darby canine kidney cells 91
Medical countermeasures 103
Medications, antiviral 127
Medicine
  integrative 100
  mainstream 225
  osteopathic 223, 224
MedImmune 63, 65, 66
Mekong Delta 157, 199
Merck 34, 63, 263
Metals, heavy 209, 211, 213, 216, 221, 222, 227
MF59 85, 95, 96-100, 269
Mice
  dioxin-exposed 277
  dioxin-laden 187
Microchips, human 120

Migratory
  birds 184, 190, 191, 193-196, 212, 214, 229, 232
  pathways 193
  patterns 193
Mills, opened pulp 229
Minor, Phil 78, 82
Molecular mimicry 97, 171, 256
Monk Gregor Mendel 171
Monkey virus 266, 268
Monsanto 138, 174, 175, 177, 178, 180, 244, 245, 283
Mortality rate 186, 239
Movie, made-for-television 47, 49
Moyers Report 226, 281
Myopic fixation 218

N
National Animal Identification System 155
National Immunization Program 1, 42, 43, 63
National Influenza Immunization Program 33
National Influenza Summit 65
National Vaccine Information Center Co-Founder 270
National Vaccine Injury Compensation Program 110-113
National Vaccine Program 25, 82, 110, 269
Netherlands 18, 89, 91, 142, 202
Neuraminidase
  enzyme 14, 122, 127, 129-131
  inhibitors 121, 122, 125, 126, 131
New Hope Group 165, 174
New Jersey Agent Orange Commission 203, 206
Newcastle's disease 171
Nigeria 229
North Sumatra 207

Other Products Available by Dr. Tenpenny

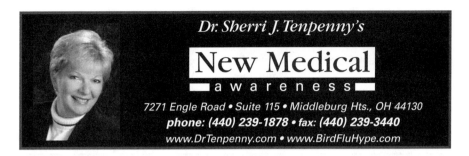

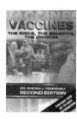

**Vaccines – The Risks, The
Benefits, The Choices DVD**
Retail Price: **$24.95**

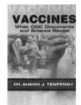

**Vaccines - What CDC Documents
& Science Reveal DVD**
Retail Price: **$24.95**

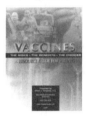

**Vaccine Resource Guide
for Parent's**
Newly updated!
Retail Price: **$34.95**

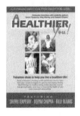

A Healthier You! Book
Retail Price: **$19.95**

**Your Body's Master Regulators:
The Thyroid/Adrenal Glands**
2-hour CD — **$14.95**

**The Link Between Food And Illness:
Eating Smart, Feeling Healthy**
2-hour CD - Live recording — **$14.95**

Osteoporosis: What Every Woman Must Know
2-hour CD — **$14.95**

ADD/ADHD/Autism: The Missing Link
2-hour CD-Live recording — **$14.95**

New Hope for Healing Fibromyalgia
2-hour CD-Live recording — **$14.95**

Introduction to Treating Vaccine Injuries
60-minute audiotape — **$12.95**
BioEnergetics Conference

Women's Breast Health
1-hour CD – **$12.95**
*Add $3.00 for corresponding printout
of powerpoint presentation

Introduction to Treating Vaccine Injuries
60-minute audiotape — **$12.95**
BioEnergetics Conference

**Menopause/Pre-menopause:
Know Your Body, Know Your Choices**
90-minute audiotape — **$12.95**

OsteoMed II's Allergy Elimination Protocol
audio CD — **$3.95**

**OsteoMed II's Approach to Treating Autism
Spectrum Disorder**
audio CD — **$3.95**

Order Form

Make checks payable to: **New Medical Awareness 7271 Engle Road, Suite 115**
                                                 Middleburg Hts., OH 44130
Order online at: **www.DrTenpenny.com**
Call or fax at: **Phone: (440) 239-1878 • Fax: (440) 239-3440**

Description	Quantity	Unit Price	Subtotal

Shipping/Handling		

Order Total	
Tax	
Shipping	
Final Total	

Shipping/Handling
CDs and DVDs ....$4.95 for 1st
and $1.50 each addt'l.
Books ....$6.95 for 1st
and $1.50 each addt'l.
Foreign shipments extra
Bulk purchases are custom quoted
Call 800-771-2147

Method of Payment
❑ MasterCard   ❑ Visa   ❑ Check

Name _____

Address _____

_____

Phone _____

Email _____

Credit Card # _____

Expiration Date _____

Signature _____